STUDENT WORKBOOK

for

DIGITAL RADIOGRAPHY IN PRACTICE

STUDENT WORKBOOK

for

DIGITAL RADIOGRAPHY IN PRACTICE

By

QUINN B. CARROLL, M.ED., R.T.

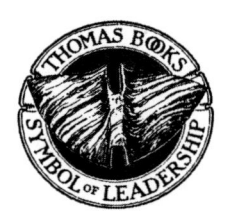

CHARLES C THOMAS • PUBLISHER, LTD.
Springfield • Illinois • U.S.A.

Published and Distributed Throughout the World by

CHARLES C THOMAS • PUBLISHER, LTD.
2600 South First Street
Springfield, Illinois 62704

This book is protected by copyright. No part of
it may be reproduced in any manner without written
permission from the publisher. All rights reserved.

© 2019 by CHARLES C THOMAS • PUBLISHER, LTD.

ISBN 978-0-398-0398-09298-6 (comb/paper)
ISBN 978-0-398-0398-09299-3 (ebook)

With THOMAS BOOKS *careful attention is given to all details of manufacturing and design. It is the Publisher's desire to present books that are satisfactory as to their physical qualities and artistic possibilities and appropriate for their particular use.* THOMAS BOOKS *will be true to those laws of quality that assure a good name and good will.*

Printed in the United States of America
MM-C-1

INTRODUCTION

How to Use this Student Workbook

The **Workbook** is entirely organized in a "fill-in-the-blank" format. The wording of each question almost exactly matches the lecture slide series <u>Digital Radiography in Practice: Instructor PowerPoint™ Slides</u>, and closely matches the progression of concepts in the textbook. The guiding philosophy is to provide immediate or short-term reinforcement of lecture and reading material by focusing on *key words*. The **Workbook** should therefore be used on a *daily basis,* not as a self-test or review after whole units have been covered. Following are specific recommendations on how the student (and instructor) can most fully benefit from the Workbook and other ancillaries to <u>Digital Radiography in Practice</u>:

1. IN-CLASS USE (RECOMMENDED):

   This is the most recommended method, for use with the **Digital Radiography in Practice Instructor PowerPoint Slides**. The workbook and slides are designed to work in tandem with each other to *actively engage* the student in classroom learning while at the same time minimizing the amount of note-taking so that the student is allowed to concentrate on the lecture. The sequence and wording of questions almost exactly matches the slides, using a fill-in-the-blank approach connected to highlighted *key words on the slides*.

   Instructors may elect to require this type of classroom use and award points for completion of each unit.

2. HOMEWORK USE:

   If the **Workbook** is used as a reinforcement tool for *homework,* it is strongly recommended that the student answer the corresponding questions after reading *each major section* of a chapter. If you wait until completing an entire chapter, you may have trouble recalling the *key words* elicited by each question and are more likely to confuse different concepts. To facilitate this, the major unit subheadings are included in the **Workbook** to match the textbook.

3. UNIT REVIEW AND SELF-TESTING:

For the purposes of review, self-testing or preparation immediately prior to a test, **Chapter Review Questions** are provided at the end of each chapter in the textbook. Answer keys to these questions may be made available from your instructor. These are better suited to unit review and test preparation than the workbook material.

CONTENTS

Page

Introduction v

Chapter
1. NATURE OF THE DIGITAL RADIOGRAPH 3
2. CREATING THE LATENT IMAGE 9
3. QUALITIES OF THE DIGITAL RADIOGRAPH 15
4. RADIOGRAPHIC TECHNIQUE FOR DIGITAL IMAGING 23
5. PREPROCESSING AND HISTOGRAM ANALYSIS 30
6. RESCALING (PROCESSING) THE DIGITAL RADIOGRAPH 38
7. DEFAULT POSTPROCESSING I: GRADATION PROCESSING 41
8. DEFAULT POSTPROCESSING II: DETAIL PROCESSING 49
9. MANIPULATING THE DIGITAL IMAGE: OPERATOR ADJUSTMENTS 56
10. MONITORING AND CONTROLLING EXPOSURE 63
11. DIGITAL IMAGE ACQUISITION 69
12. DISPLAYING THE DIGITAL IMAGE 88
13. ARCHIVING PATIENT IMAGES AND INFORMATION 97
14. DIGITAL FLUOROSCOPY 105
15. QUALITY CONTROL FOR DIGITAL EQUIPMENT 114

STUDENT WORKBOOK

for

DIGITAL RADIOGRAPHY IN PRACTICE

Chapter 1

NATURE OF THE DIGITAL RADIOGRAPH

Development of Digital Radiography

1. 1979—First application of digital tech: Digital _____ unit.

2. 1982—PACS and _____.

3. 1980s—Computed radiography (CR): Initially led to a _____ of exposure.

4. 1996—Digital radiography (DR): Advanced miniaturization of _____ elements.

5. For CR, x-ray energy stored by a phosphor is emitted as _____ when stimulated by a laser beam.

6. For direct-conversion DR, x-ray energy is converted directly into stored _____ charge.

7. For indirect-conversion DR, a _____ first converts x-rays to light, then the light is converted into electrical charge.

8. All CR and DR systems ultimately produce an _____ image signal that is "fed" into a computer for processing.

Nature of the Digital Image

9. All forms of digital image acquisition result in an image _____.

10. Each _____ (picture element) is a single location designated by its column and row.

11. Each pixel is assigned a pixel value that will become its _____ upon display.

12. Light images enter a camera, and x-rays enter a detector, in _____ form.

13. To manipulate these images with a computer, they must first be converted into _____ form.

14. Analog: Continuous, and infinitely _____, like the rails of a railroad track.

15. Digital: Discrete (separated into _____ units), limited in subdivision and in scale, like the wooden ties of a railroad track.

16. Mathematically, digitization means _____ all measurements to the nearest available digital value in a pre-set scale.

17. This rounding out makes digital information *inherently* less _____ than analog information.

18. However, as long as the discrete units for a digital computer are smaller than the human eye can detect, digitizing the information improves _____ accuracy.

19. This is why _____ equipment is used to clock the winner of a race in the Olympics.

20. Rounding these input values (A) out to the nearest allowable discrete unit (B) so the computer can manage them is the function of an _____-to-_____ converter (ADC).

Digitizing the Analog Image

21. Three Steps to Digitizing the Image: 1. _____
    2. _____
    3. _____

22. Scanning: Image is divided up into a(n) _____ of pixel cells.

23. Sampling: _____ of light (or x-rays) is measured for each cell.

24. Scanning: In CR, the reader (processor) is set to scan the PSP plate in a pre-designated number of _____, and samplings per _____.

25. In DR (and DF using CCDs), since the number of available pixels is the number of detector elements (dexels) embedded in the image receptor plate, collimation of the x-ray beam is analogous to _____.

26. Sampling Aperture: Opening through which _____ are taken.

27. DR: Sampling aperture determined by _____ _____ (dexels) in the IR, which are square in shape and do not overlap adjacent samplings.

28. CR: Sampling aperture determined by reading _____ beam in CR reader, which is circular in shape, overlapping adjacent samplings that must then be "cropped."

29. Quantizing: Discrete numerical value is assigned to each cell from a pre-designated _____ _____.

Bit Depth, Dynamic Range, and Gray Scale

30. The terms bit depth and dynamic range are often used interchangeably by physicists and _____, which can be confusing for the student. For clarity, we will define them according to their most dominant use by experts.

31. Bit Depth: The maximum range of pixel values a computer, display monitor, DR detector or other _____ device can store, expressed as an exponent of base 2.

    "6 bits deep" = $2^{—}$ = 64 values
    "7 bits deep" = $2^{—}$ = 128 values
    "8 bits deep" = 2^{8} = ____ values

32. The human eye can only discern about $2^{—}$ = ___ shades of gray or levels of brightness (a bit depth of __).

33. By not using the full range of bit depth of the computer, image processing _____ can be accelerated.

34. Dynamic range compression _____ off the extreme ends of the bit depth that are not needed to construct images, to save processing speed. This does not affect the displayed image.

35. Dynamic Range: The range of pixel values (from the bit depth) that the entire system makes _____ to build up images.

36. Dynamic range is determined by _____ as well as hardware.

37. Dynamic range is also the number of gray shades with which each _____ can be represented by the system.

38. Gray Scale: The range of pixel values actually present in a _____ image.

39. Dynamic range is a _____ of Bit Depth. Gray Scale is a subset of _____ _____.

40. The greater the dynamic range, the _____ the gray scale in the displayed image.

41. The longer the gray scale, the more _____ can be represented in the image.

42. Excessive dynamic range _____ down image processing time. Insufficient dynamic range causes loss of image _____.

43. Insufficient dynamic range prevents full post _____ capabilities for the image:

44. We must be able to double or cut in half both the brightness and contrast of the image _____ times without running out of dynamic range (data clipping). Complex features such as subtraction require still more.

45. The dynamic range of the remnant x-ray beam is approximately 2—.

46. The enhanced contrast resolution and processing features of CT and MRI systems require a ____-bit deep range.

Nature of the Digital Radiograph

47. Most digital imaging systems have dynamic ranges set at $2^8 = 256$, $2^{10} = 1024$ (___ and ___), or $2^{12} = 4048$.

What is a Pixel?

48. To a computer expert, a pixel has no particular shape or dimensions - It is a point location or _____ which has been assigned a numerical value.

49. For displayed medical images, however, we define a pixel as the _____ screen element which can represent all gray levels within the dynamic range of the imaging system.

50. These elements do have both a shape and an area _____.

51. For the radiographer, it is best to visualize pixels as generally _____ in shape and having a set size.

52. For an LCD display monitor, each hardware pixel is formed by the _____ of two flat, transparent wires. Their dimensions are typically ___mm square.

Voxels, Dexels and Pixels

53. Attenuation Coefficient: The _____ or _____ of original x-ray beam intensity absorbed by a particular tissue area in the patient.

54. The attenuation coefficient is determined by data acquired from 3-dimensional volumes of tissue within the patient called _____, an acronym for "_____-elements."

55. Each _____ in a radiographic image represents a voxel within the patient.

56. CT scanners can isolate a 3-D cube of tissue because they combine multiple _____ from hundreds of angles.

57. Since DR and CR only use a single projection, the 3-D voxels sampled are in the shape of long, square tubes that pass from the _____ to the _____ of the patient.

58. To assign a gray level to a pixel in the final image, within each voxel the attenuation coefficients for various tissues must be _____.

59. These attenuation coefficients must then be rounded out by the ADC to _____ values from the system's dynamic range.

60. The ultimate brightness of each pixel brought up on the display monitor is controlled by the amount of electrical voltage applied to it, which depends on the _____ _____ number stored in the computer for that pixel.

61. We might say that to form a digital radiographic image, data from the _____ in the patient are collected by the dexels of the image receptor, then computer processed to become the _____ of the displayed image.

Chapter 2

CREATING THE LATENT IMAGE

Overview of Variables

1. Latent Image: Information carried by the _____ x-ray beam to the image receptor

2. List the three general types of radiographic variables for the latent Image:
   _____
   _____
   _____

3. Give two examples for each of the three general types of radiographic variables for the latent Image:
   _____ _____
   _____ _____
   _____ _____

4. X-ray absorption by air is _____, less than ___% of the geometrical effect of the inverse square law.

5. Nearly ALL the effect of increased SID is due to the simple _____ of the inverse square law.

6. Within the patient, _____ interactions are primarily responsible for production of subject contrast in the remnant x-ray beam.

7. Compton and Thompson interactions generate scatter radiation and are _____ to subject contrast.

8. Attenuation: The _____ absorption of x-rays by body tissues.

9. Attenuation is essential to production of an image _____ in the remnant x-ray beam.

10. Without attenuation, rather than various shades of gray representing different tissues, a silhouette image would result with little _____ in it.

Creating Subject Contrast

11. Within the patient, photoelectric Interactions are primarily responsible for creating _____ shades.

12. Compton scatter: Responsible for ___% of all scatter radiation.

13. Thompson scatter produces only 2–3% of _____ radiation.

14. Characteristic interactions result only in low-energy ultraviolet rays that do not _____ the patient's body.

Of Primary Interest for radiographic technique:

15. Penetrating X-rays: Responsible for creating subject contrast (_____).

16. Photoelectric Interactions: Responsible for creating subject contrast (_____).

17. Compton Scatter: Mostly responsible for destroying subject contrast by adding "fog" to the latent image reaching the _____ _____.

18. In the remnant x-ray beam, the useful signal is created by variations in the photoelectric/penetration _____ for different tissues of the body.

19. Compton Scatter carries no useful signal, but is a _____-distributed form of noise that hinders visibility of the useful image.

20. A "hardened" x-ray beam with higher _____ energy can be created by either increasing the set kVp OR by adding filtration.

21. kVp is the primary controlling factor for x-ray beam _____.

22. As average x-ray beam energy is increased, ALL x-rays have increased _____ of penetration.

Creating the Latent Image 11

23. Therefore, _____ types of interactions within the patient's body decrease in probability.

24. However, as x-ray beam energy (keV) increases, the probability of photoelectric interactions _____.

25. While . . . the probability of Compton interactions only decreases slightly (<___%).

26. At 80 keV, in *bone* there are still more _____ occurring than Comptons, creating good subject contrast.

27. In soft tissue, however, photoelectrics have mostly _____, leaving only Compton scatter and penetrating x-rays.

28. For this reason, at 80 keV soft tissues show up _____ while bone is still demonstrated with subject contrast.

29. As the part becomes thicker, all types of interactions increase by equal _____.

30. For every 4–5 cm increase in part thickness, radiographic technique must be _____.

31. Physical density is the _____ of mass.

32. As the number of molecules per volume, density can be changed by _____.

33. Tissue density is directly proportional to general attenuation. Therefore, it is directly proportional to the needed radiographic _____.

34. High atomic number (Z#) means that the atom also has many more electrons concentrated into about the same space, called the "electron _____."

35. This makes it much more likely that an x-ray will strike an _____ electron.

36. X-ray absorption increases by the _____ of the atomic number. Example, carbon is 6 x 6 x 6 = 216 times more likely to absorb an x-ray than hydrogen.

37. This is the main reason _____ contrast agents, such as Iodine and Barium, work so well absorbing x-rays.

38. Iodine Z# = ____
    Barium Z# = ____
    Soft Tissue Effective Z# = ____

39. Using the Z-cubed relationship, we find that positive contrast agents are approximately ____ times more effective at X-ray absorption than soft tissue.

40. Air Effective Z# = ____
    Soft Tissue Effective Z# = ____, nearly equal, but . . .
    Air density = ~ 1/_____th that of soft tissue.

41. Negative contrast agents are gasses, and work primarily due to their _____ difference in physical density.
    (See textbook discussion for bone vs. soft tissue.)

42. List the 5 main variables affecting subject contrast in the remnant x-ray beam:

43. Subject contrast is determined by the distribution or _____ of different types of interactions taking place within the patient.

44. mAs is _____ a controlling factor for subject contrast:

45. At twice the mAs, there are twice as many penetrating x-rays, twice as many photoelectrics, and twice as many Comptons. All interactions change by the same _____. The distribution or ratio of different interactions remains unchanged.

46. SID is ____ a controlling factor for subject contrast:

47. At 3/4 the SID (due to the inverse square law), again, all interactions change by the same proportion. Therefore . . . the distribution or ratio of different interactions remains _____.

48. At the image receptor, both mAs and SID change the overall intensity of exposure, but NOT the _____ of different types of interactions.

49. It is possible for an image to be twice as dark, yet still have the same _____.

50. Neither mAs nor SID should be considered as _____ factors for subject contrast.

Role of Radiographic Technique in the Digital Age

51. To simply provide _____ signal reaching the IR, enough information for the computer to process.

52. This depends on both beam _____ controlled by mAs and SID, AND beam _____ controlled by filtration and kVp.

53. This allows great leeway in employing _____-kVp techniques to reduce patient dose when the mAs is compensated according to the 15% rule.

Subject Contrast and Sharpness

54. The image signal is carried by the _____ x-ray beam.

55. It possesses:
    Subject contrast
    Noise in the form of scatter radiation and quantum _____.
    Inherent _____, magnification and distortion determined by beam geometry and positioning.

56. This is NOT the final image _____ on a monitor.
    That image will be radically altered in nearly every way by digital _____.

57. The remnant beam signal does set important _____ on what digital processing can do.

58. There must be a minimum level of _____ subject contrast.

59. However, this is an extremely minor requirement in practice, because digital processing has ____ times the contrast enhancement capability of film technology.

60. This high contrast enhancement allows us to use high kVp techniques to reduce _____ dose.

61. Sharpness is of more concern in the _____ age.

62. A typical display monitor has a hardware pixel size of ____ mm.

63. At typical SID, the SOD/OID ratio results in an "effective pixel size" comparable to the display _____.

64. This means that in some circumstances, using the large focal spot when the small FS should be used could cause more _____ than the display monitor.

65. Good x-ray beam geometry is still important, and the _____ focal spot should be used whenever feasible, especially with distal extremities.

66. Variables Affecting Quality of Final Displayed Image:
    Characteristics of the IR—Chapter 11
    Digital Processing—Chapters 5 through 10
    Characteristics of the Display Monitor—Chapter 12
    Ambient Viewing Conditions—Chapters 12 and 15

Chapter 3

QUALITIES OF THE DIGITAL RADIOGRAPH

Qualities of the Final Displayed Digital Image

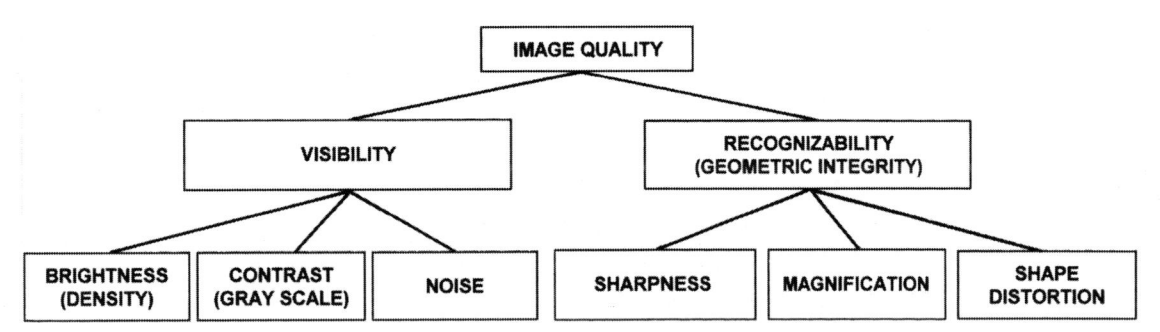

Figure 3.1. Hierarchy of Displayed Image Qualities.

1. The six fundamental image qualities combine into _____ and _____ factors to produce overall image quality.

2. Brightness refers to the _____ of light for any portion of the image.

3. The ideal level of brightness is an _____ level in which all pixels within the anatomy of interest are displayed as a level of gray, neither blank white nor pitch black.

4. Strictly speaking, as shown on the CT scans, when "leveling," increasing window Level makes a radiographic image _____.

5. Window level is the opposite of brightness: Increasing brightness brings the level number _____.

6. Density: The _____ of any portion of the image. (Still used especially for hard copies of radiographic images.)

7. Optical density is measured as the opposite of _____, but conveys the same concept.

8. Again, ideal overall density is _____, (neither minimum nor maximum).

9. Contrast: Defined as the _____ or _____ between the brightness of two adjacent areas of the image.

10. A certain minimum contrast is necessary for _____.

11. Gray Scale: Defined as the _____ of different brightness levels (or densities) within an image.

12. Long gray scale presents _____ shades of gray. Short gray scale has only a few different shades, counted on a scale from white to black.

13. Gray scale is associated with the amount of _____ present in the image.

14. The more shades of gray available, the more different types of _____ can be demonstrated.

15. Generally, gray scale is considered the _____ of contrast.

16. Progressing from black to white, when more shades of gray are present, there must be less _____ between one step and the next.

17. With too long gray scale, there can be too little _____ between details, such that it is difficult to tell them apart.

18. Strictly speaking, as shown on the CT scans, when "windowing," increasing window width gives a radiographic image more _____ _____.

19. Window width is the _____ of contrast: Increasing the contrast brings the window number down.

20. Generally, ideal level of contrast or gray scale is optimum, an _____ level, (not maximum nor minimum).

21. Contrast must always be measured between tissues within the _____—not between the pitch-black background density and a tissue.

22. (Although at very extreme levels of underexposure or overexposure, contrast can be destroyed, this is the _____, not the rule: There is a wide range of exposures within which the image can be darkened or lightened without contrast being affected.

23. To calculate contrast, always use a ratio or percentage (_____) rather than subtraction.

24. Example: Starting with two densities measuring 1 and 2: Add a fog density of 1
    Using Subtraction: Original contrast = _____
                         New contrast = _____
                         Conclusion: Fog has NOT altered contrast = FALSE

25. Using Division: Original contrast = _____
                         New contrast = _____
                         Conclusion: Fog has reduced contrast = TRUE

26. Image **noise** is defined as any non-useful contribution to the image that interferes with the _____ of anatomy or pathology of interest.

27. Dr. Anthony Wolbarst's The Physics of Radiology: "Noise is _____ in an image that detracts from its clinical usefulness."

28. The "ideal" level of noise is always _____.

29. List the 8 general types of image noise:
    1. _____
    2. _____
    3. _____
    4. _____
    5. _____
    6. _____
    7. _____
    8. _____

30. In the digital age, image _____ has far exceeded "fog" from scatter radiation as the most common form of noise appearing in the final displayed image.

31. Some authors have restricted the meaning of noise to only quantum mottle, but this is misleading—For example, there are also four types of _____ mottle.

32. Scatter radiation is also a form of noise, as are various artifacts that interfere with _____ of important diagnostic details

33. Scatter radiation and off-_____ radiation are both forms of noise that are destructive to image contrast.

34. Exposure artifacts include _____ lines, extraneous objects, and false images such as tomographic streaks.

35. Aliasing artifacts (Chap. 11) are _____ line patterns very common with electronically displayed digital images.

36. Even "algorithmic noise" can be caused by imperfections in image reconstruction _____.

37. Background fluctuations, surges and dips in electrical current which are present in any electronic system, are classified as _____ noise in the image.

38. Electronic "snow" is also common in _____.

39. Signal-to-Noise Ratio (SNR) is a measure of the overall _____ of information.

40. The signal refers to all of the _____, useful information carried by the subject contrast in the remnant x-ray beam.
    Penetrated dark shades
    Attenuated medium shades
    Absorbed light shades

41. The noise consists of all forms of destructive, non-_____ input.

42. Defined as the proportion of all useful diagnostic information to all obstructing _____.

43. SNR is a _____ number useful in comparing images.

Qualities of the Digital Radiograph   19

44. Two ways to improve SNR:
    – Reduce noise
    – Increase signal (x-ray intensity reaching the IR, either by _____ [kVp] or original _____ [mAs].

45. Example: Improving SNR by reducing noise: With a relative signal of 3, decreasing the noise from 2 to 1:
    Original SNR: $\frac{S}{N} = \frac{3}{2} = 1.5$
    New SNR: $\frac{S}{N} = \frac{3}{1} = $ _____

46. Example: Improving SNR by increasing signal: With a relative noise of 2, increasing the signal from 3 to 4:
    Original SNR: $\frac{S}{N} = \frac{3}{2} = 1.5$
    New SNR: $\frac{S}{N} = \frac{4}{2} = $ _____

47. Sharpness of detail is defined as the _____ with which the edges of an image "stop."

48. While moving across the image, if the edge of a detail suddenly changes from white to the black background, (A) the image is _____.

49. While moving across the image, if the edge of a detail _____ changes to the background density, the image is unsharp.

50. Sharpness is affected by the focal spot, beam projection _____ and any motion during exposure.

51. _____ sharpness is always the goal.

52. Shape Distortion is defined as the difference between the shape of a real object and the shape of it _____ image.

53. In radiography, shape distortion is caused by _____ of the x-ray tube, the body part, or the image receptor. This includes off-angling and off-centering.

54. Shape distortion is the one image quality that _____ processing does not alter!

20   *Student Workbook for Digital Radiography in Practice*

55. Geometric Magnification (also referred to as size distortion), is defined as the difference between the size of a real object and the size of its _____ image.

56. Geometric magnification can simulate a _____ condition, and lead to diagnostic misinformation, (such as inaccurate heart size).

57. Magnification Technique: Can be used _____ in some cases (such as in angiography, when an aneurism or blood clot are too small to recognize).

58. Display Magnification is a change in size created by applying "zoom" or "magnify" features of a display monitor, or by any form of post-collimation that changes the _____-___-_____ within the physical area of the monitor screen.

59. Certain levels of excessive magnification can result in:
   1. A "_____" image
   2. Aliasing patterns (Moire artifact)

60. Brightness, contrast, and noise combine to determine the _____ of an image.

61. Sharpness, shape distortion and magnification make up the _____ (geometrical integrity) of the image.

62. Qualities of the Latent Image captured at the Image Receptor include:
   _____ intensity
   Subject contrast
   Noise
   Inherent sharpness from beam projection geometry
   Shape distortion
   Geometrical magnification

63. These are NOT to be confused with qualities of the FINAL _____ IMAGE.

64. ALL except _____ distortion are altered by digital processing.

Comparison of Latent Image qualities to Displayed Image qualities:

65. In the *latent image,* what do we have in place of "brightness":

Qualities of the Digital Radiograph 21

66. In the *displayed image,* what two types of noise and sharpness are *added* to "original noise and sharpness":

67. In the *displayed image,* what type of magnification is *added* to geometrical magnification:

68. Quoting the AAPM (American Association of Physicists in Medicine), "Image display in digital radiography is _____ of image acquisition."

69. "Qualities of the final displayed image are _____ from conditions of the original x-ray exposure."

70. At the microscopic level, *resolution* is specifically defined as the ability to distinguish two adjacent details as being _____ from each other.

71. When comparing the *resolution* capability of two different imaging systems, physicists are primarily concerned with resolving a single ____ or _____, whereas the radiographer is concerned with the true representation of a bone or other anatomical structure.

72. Physicists analyze the image at the microscopic level. Radiographers evaluate the image at the clinical (_____) level.

73. For the physicist, at the microscopic level the image has only two qualities: _____ Resolution and _____ Resolution.

74. At the microscopic level, the only two questions are: "Can you make out the dot against the _____ and _____ from other dots?"

75. On the radiographers' hierarchy of image qualities, *Contrast Resolution* best correlates to overall _____.

76. On the radiographers' hierarchy of image qualities, *Spatial Resolution* best correlates to overall _____ (Geometrical Integrity).

77. The six qualities apply to a _____, not to a dot . . . e.g., a single dot cannot contain "noise" or "distortion."

78. For a single detail (dot, or line), the exposure trace diagram can represent the contrast of the detail as the vertical _____ of the "pit."

79. For a single detail (dot, or line), the exposure trace diagram can represent the blur (penumbra) as the horizontal _____ of the slopes. For the physicist, these correlate to contrast resolution and spatial resolution.

80. When a resolution template is exposed, the projection of several thin lead strips and slits results in a series of density trace diagrams that begin to look like a sine _____.

81. Modulation Transfer Function (MTF) is defined as the ability of an imaging system to _____ modulating (oscillating) densities (black/white/black/white) to the displayed image in the form of thin lines or dots.

82. In the resulting wave form, the rounding of corners in the diagram represents _____.

83. As lines become smaller and closer together, eventually overlapping penumbras cause a decline in the vertical dimension of the sine wave, representing reduced _____ at the microscopic level.

84. Resolution template images show that overall resolution can be lost by either blurred edges resulting in poor _____ even though contrast is high, or by poor _____ even though sharpness is high.

Chapter 4

RADIOGRAPHIC TECHNIQUE FOR DIGITAL IMAGING

1. In the digital age, the new role for set radiographic technique is to provide _____ signal at the image receptor for the computer to be able to manipulate the data.

2. We desire maximum _____ information (signal) with minimum noise to achieve maximum signal/noise ratio (SNR).

3. As with conventional radiography, to provide sufficient SNR, it is still true that no amount of intensity can compensate for inadequate _____.

4. No amount of _____ can compensate for inadequate kVp.

Understanding X-Ray Beam Penetration

5. Sufficient x-ray penetration is essential for adequate _____ to reach the image receptor.

6. *Penetration* is generally defined as the _____ or ratio of x-rays that make it through the patient, tabletop and grid to strike the IR.

7. All the IR "cares about" is its _____ exposure level from the *remnant* x-ray beam, not the specific intensity of the primary beam.

8. Total exposure at the IR is not based on the mAs alone, but on the _____ of kVp and mAs used.

9. If penetration is doubled at a higher kVp, then ____ the mAs can be used to achieve equal dose to the IR.

Sensitivity of Digital Units to Subject Contrast

10. Subject Contrast is the ratio between adjacent areas of the remnant x-ray beam representing different _____ within the body.

11. Subject contrast is produced by differences in part thickness, effective atomic number, and physical _____ of different tissues.

12. For any image, a _____ level of subject contrast must be present to distinguish between tissue areas.

13. A CT scanner is able to distinguish between gray matter and white matter in brain tissue, and display the eyeballs within periorbital fat. A conventional radiograph is only able to demonstrate _____, _____, and _____ generally.

14. Computerized (digital) imaging is more _____ to the original subject contrast of the incoming remnant beam image.

15. Conventional film imaging required a minimum 10% subject contrast to distinguish between tissues. Digital imaging requires only ___% subject contrast, because of its contrast-enhancing capabilities.

16. Digital technology provides ___X the contrast resolution of film technology!

Subject Contrast and Exposure Latitude

17. Exposure Latitude is defined as the range of radiographic _____ that can produce an acceptable image.

18. Exposure latitude is also the margin for _____ in setting technique.

19. This margin for error includes use of different _____, filters, focal spots, and distances.

20. Generally, a latent image possessing higher subject contrast will present _____ exposure latitude.

21. High contrast (short gray scale) allows less _____ to move the displayed densities (solid arrow) up or down the available dynamic range.

22. Lengthened gray scale allows greater changes in technique without "running out" of available _____.

23. Since digital systems require only 1% subject contrast, the result is a much extended _____ _____. There is _____ margin for technique error.

24. All technical aspects of the original exposure become _____ critical.

25. One result is the _____ to use grids and filters less, lower grid ratios, higher kVp's, etc.

26. However, the increased exposure latitude of digital systems extends primarily in an _____ direction.

27. On reducing technique, if exposure levels at the IR reach less than 1/3 ideal exposure, the appearance of _____ is certain.

28. For increases in technique, the only restricting factor is the effect on _____ dose. (Normally, there are no noticeable effects on the displayed image.)

Reducing Use of Grids

29. Increased exposure latitude of digital systems allow flexibility to use _____–_____ techniques for some procedures that used to require grids.

30. Increased exposure latitude of digital systems allow flexibility to use _____ grid ratios for procedures that still require a grid.

31. Both of these practices allow less mAs to be used, reducing _____ _____.

32. Non-grid technique requires ____ or less mAs to be used, reducing patient dose to this amount.

33. Using a 6:1 grid ratio instead of 10:1 or 12:1 allows mAs to be cut in _____, reducing patient dose to this amount.

34. By reducing grid use, some scatter radiation is allowed "back" into the beam, BUT digital processing routinely restores nearly all the "damage" done by moderate amounts of _____.

35. Digital systems only require 1% subject contrast. If subject contrast is reduced from 10% to 5%, the system can still _____ for it.

36. Only the most _____ cases of scatter show up on display.

37. _____ forms of noise increase the risk of digital processing errors.

38. Using a grid reduces noise in the form of scatter. However, if the technique is not compensated, removing a grid reduces the probability of noise in the form of _____.

39. Which is more important to remove? Reducing patient dose and the probability of mottle can _____ be achieved:

40. First, remove the grid. By removing a 10:1 or 12:1 table bucky grid, one-_____ of the mAs could be used. This would result in a 75% reduction in patient dose.

41. Second, reduce the _____ only to 1/2 or 1/3 of the original grid technique, (instead of 1/4).

42. The image receptor is now receiving more radiation than the grid technique allowed, such that _____ is less likely, yet patient dose has also been cut by ____–____% from the grid technique!

43. Several manufacturers now offer _____ grid software that replaces the need for grids except in the most extreme circumstances, (such as abdominal projections on obese patients).

44. Evaluation of several manufacturers virtual grid software shows it to be about ____% as effective as conventional grids.

Compared to conventional grid use, with *virtual grid* software:

45. The effects of _____ are increased slightly,

46. The likelihood of _____ appearing is reduced.

47. Risk of grid cut-off is _____, allowing more flexibility in positioning, especially for trauma and mobile procedures.

48. Radiation exposure to the patient is _____.

Even if conventional grids continue in use, the following are strongly recommended:

49. Consider non-grid techniques at least for these 5 types of procedures:
    _____
    _____
    _____
    _____
    _____

50. Use a 6:1 grid ratio for all gridded _____ procedures.

51. Reduce grid ratio to ____ in all fixed units, and reduce mAs values accordingly.

52. Grids should not be used when it is _____.

53. Digital technology is allowing us as a profession to explore and adopt tools that will benefit the _____ in various ways.

Sufficient Input Gray Scale

54. Starting with a long-scale input image, if shortened gray scale is desired, the computer can select every-other density. In this case, all final displayed information consists of _____ values measured at the IR.

55. Starting with a short-scale input image, if lengthened gray scale is desired, the computer must extrapolate new values. In this case, new values are _____ and constitute _____ information.

56. Generally, for digital radiography, long gray scale in the latent image is _____ because it provides more real tissue information.

57. Long gray scale in the latent image is primarily achieved through the use of _____ kVp techniques.

Minimizing Patient Exposure with the 15% Rule

58. Cutting the mAs in half results in ____ exposure at the IR (and for the patient).

59. A 15% increase in kVp restores exposure to the IR for two reasons: First, increased penetration through the patient recovers about _____ of the exposure to the IR.

60. Second, higher kVp results in ~35% more bremsstrahlung x-rays being produced in the x-ray tube. This recovers an additional _____ of the original exposure to the IR.

61. The combined effect is that exposure to the IR is _____.

At the surface of the patient:

62. Cutting the mAs in half reduces patient exposure to ____%.

63. The increase in kVp adds back about ____% from increased bremsstrahlung production.

64. 35% of 50 = 17, 50 + 17 = ____ percent final count.

65. Applying the 15% rule reduces patient dose to about 2/3 the original exposure. Patient dose is cut by ____.

At the Image receptor:

66. Now, the aspect of _____ enters into the equation.

67. For example, assume that from 80 to 92 kVp, penetration increases from 6.7% TO 10%. 6.7% of 1000 = 67. 10% of 670 = 67. Exposure to the IR is fully _____ to 67.

68. The *end result* of cutting mAs in half and increasing kVp 15% is that patient dose was reduced from 1000 x-rays to 670 x-rays (67%), while exposure to the ___ was maintained.

Benefits of High-kVp Radiography

69. High kVp helps ensure sufficient x-ray _____ through the patient to the IR.

70. High kVp provides long gray scale _____ to the computer for manipulation without interpolation.

71. High kVp reduces _____ exposure when combined with lower mAs values.

72. For digital systems, the overall reduction in image contrast is visually _____ for each 15% step increase in kVp, (proven for nine different manufacturers).

73. With digital systems, even a 52-kVp increase demonstrates only the expected lengthening of gray scale due to increased penetration. There is no _____ pattern in these high-kVp digital images (as there would be with film).

74. In addition, digital software can identify and correct for expected fog _____ such as those encountered on the lateral lumbar spine projection.

A study of nine manufacturers' digital equipment showed that:

75. Generally, it took three 15% step-increases to show a _____ increase in mottle.

76. Mottle was _____ significant for a single-step application of the 15 percent rule.

77. Departments can apply a single 15% increase in kVp, and cut mAs in half, across the board for ____ techniques.

Chapter 5

PREPROCESSING AND HISTOGRAM ANALYSIS

1. All methods of capturing information from the remnant x-ray beam involve the _____ of atoms or molecules.

2. For film, ionization led to chemical changes that darkened the film. For digital radiography, electrons "freed" by ionization are _____ up on a capacitor.

3. The amount of charge is measured and recorded as a _____ value number.

4. All these numbers together make up the _____ set that will be processed by a computer.

The Generic Steps of Digital Image Processing

5. Conventional film processing consisted of 4 steps: Chemical developing, chemical fixing, washing, and drying. These steps had to be followed in _____.

6. Digital image processing consists of at least 9 steps. They are applied in _____ order by different manufacturers.

7. For digital processing, some steps (such as noise reduction) are even _____ at different stages of processing.

8. *Preprocessing* (Acquisition Processing) refers to all *corrections* made to the "raw" digital image data to compensate for physical _____ in image acquisition inherent in the elements and circuitry of the image receptor, and physical elements and circuitry of the processor.

9. The "raw" digital image from the IR is both very noisy and so extremely "washed out" (low contrast) that it cannot be used for _____.

10. Preprocessing and rescaling must compensate for these flaws in image _____ to make the image diagnostic.

11. *Postprocessing* refers to all adjustments (whether by default settings in the processor or by the user at the console) made after acquisition corrections have been made, targeted at _____ of the image, and somewhat subject to personal preference.

12. While preprocessing makes corrections targeted at image acquisition, *postprocessing* makes refinements targeted at the specific anatomical _____.

13. List the four generic steps of *preprocessing:*
    _____
    _____
    _____
    _____

14. List the five generic steps of *postprocessing:*
    _____
    _____
    _____
    _____
    _____

15. The first *seven* steps listed above collectively make up _____ processing which brings the image to initial display.

16. Specifically, it is _____ that gives the digital image the contrast necessary for diagnosis.

17. Rescaling is the step that best fits the concept of _____ the image—It "normalizes" the appearance of the initially displayed image.

18. However, since digital rescaling is correcting for flaws in image acquisition, it also falls under the category of _____.

Preprocessing

19. *Segmentation* software scans across the receptor plate to determine the number of views taken, and where their borders are so they are not processed together as a _____ image.

20. With segmentation failure, "blank" spaces between fields are interpreted as if they were bones or metallic objects within the body part. Averaging all densities between different exposures, the result is a final image that is _____ and low-contrast.

21. Since DR units allow only _____ exposure at a time to be processed, the segmentation step is unnecessary.

22. In DR systems, dead detector elements (dexels) can result from _____ failure of switching transistors.

23. The computer uses _____ reduction software to eliminate these "dead" spots in the image.

24. The most common way to correct these is using a software _____: The values of the 8 pixels surrounding a dead pixel are averaged, then this value is inserted into the dead pixel.

25. This process is called _____.

26. A *kernel* is defined as a ____-_____ that is passed over the larger image matrix executing some mathematical function.

27. Software can compensate for moderate cases of dexel drop-out, but not for _____ cases where whole sections of rows have dropped out.

28. There are two general types of mottle: _____ mottle and _____ mottle. When severe, the two types can be indistinguishable from each other at the gross observational level.

29. Quantum mottle appears as _____ mottle—artifacts of variable size that occur in an _____, chaotic distribution.

30. Electronic mottle appears as _____ mottle—artifacts that tend to be of consistent size and occur in a pattern at regular _____.

31. All electronics have small "microcurrent" _____ that occur naturally from various causes (e.g., local magnetic fields or natural radiation).

32. Like a light rain shower, *quantum mottle* can be seen to follow a "Poisson distribution," that is randomly distributed and of varying ____.

33. With lots of signal present, the randomness is still there, but is ____ apparent, eventually disappearing visually.

34. Digital processing can correct for _____ amounts of mottle.

35. Frequency processing is ideal for removing electronic and other _____ mottle.

36. Frequency filtering algorithms "attack" a very narrowly-defined _____ of mottle.

37. Normal anatomy has many _____ sizes, so it occurs at various frequencies.

38. Therefore, frequency processing can eliminate the image _____ containing most of the electronic mottle without affecting normal anatomy very much.

39. _____ work better for suppressing random mottle.

40. Kernels can "attack" a broader range of _____ of mottle, such as occur from the random distribution of x-rays in the beam.

41. Frequency processing generally fails to fully _____ random mottle from the image.

42. Variations in _____ uniformity are due to electronic and optical flaws in the image receptor and reader.

43. DR systems typically undergo _____ preprocessing than CR systems.

44. Examples of system *noise* include dark noise and dexel drop-out. Dark noise includes background exposure to a CR phosphor plate and dark _____ (background _____ in a DR detector system.

45. Several electronic and optical flaws result in _____ distribution of x-rays across the field.

46. The anode heel effect also contributes, but cannot be _____ compensated for.

47. Flat field uniformity corrections even out the _____ across the area of the field.

48. Field uniformity is tested using low exposure with ____ object in the field.

49. Compiling the Histogram Is simply a matter of _____ the number of pixels holding each gray level.

50. This is analogous to collecting pixels of different shades and sorting them into buckets representing computer _____.

51. The histogram is really a _____ graph indicating the number of pixels counted for each value (gray level).

52. (The histogram gives no indication of the _____ of these pixels or what anatomy they represent.)

53. The histogram is usually displayed as a "best-fit line" connecting the _____ of the bars.

Histogram Analysis

54. The histogram is based on a simple scale of _____ (or density).

55. This scale usually proceeds from _____ to _____ as read left to right, (although this scale can be reversed).

56. Histograms acquire generally consistent _____ for different body parts.

57. The key distinction between histogram types is the number of _____ (high points) generated within the data set.

58. The most common type of histogram has 2 lobes, the main lobe representing tissues within the anatomy, and the tail lobe representing "raw" _____ exposure.

59. A histogram for an image with no background density is expected to have only ___ lobe.

Preprocessing and Histogram Analysis 35

60. Expected histogram for a mammogram normally shows __ lobes.

61. The initial purpose of histogram analysis is to eliminate _____ data that will skew the rescaling of the image, making it turn out too dark or too light.

62. For rescaling to work properly, all data must represent densities within the _____ part.

63. Exposure Field Recognition (EFR) identifies the "raw" background exposure ("_____ spike") for elimination.

64. To identify the "tail spike," the computer must identify the landmark _____.

65. Several mathematical _____ can be used to identify histogram landmarks.

66. In a simplified example subtracting the number of pixels in each "bin" from the bin to the right, S_{MAX} can be identified as the second point in the data, from right to left, that _____ results occur.

67. To identify histogram landmarks, the computer scans the data _____ from both the left and the right ends of the histogram.

68. From each end, the first bin containing a ____-_____ pixel count is identified.

69. The 1st point identified at the left will be _____.

70. The goal is for all data between S_{MIN} and S_{MAX} to represent _____ structures.

71. S_{MAX} represents the _____ density within the body part.

72. At the control console, selecting the procedure algorithm assigns the type of histogram _____ to be used.

73. Each type of histogram analysis "expects" a particular shape and _____ of lobes for the acquired histogram.

74. These must _____ to avoid errors in rescaling and the EI.

75. For Type I analysis, the computer algorithm "expects" a _____ exposure area background) to be present, creating a "spike" to the right in the acquired histogram.

76. Type III analysis "expects" a large area of _____ exposure due to the presence of barium or other metal (lead shield or prosthesis), creating a "spike" to the left.

77. To accentuate particular anatomy, a computer algorithm can select a narrower range of densities from the image to operate on, called the _____ of interest (VOI).

78. Histogram Analysis Errors Can occur from several causes:
    –From _____ or exposure field recognition errors
    –When the type of histogram analysis applied is _____ to the actual histogram acquired
    –When the acquired histogram attains a bizarre, unexpected _____

79. The acquired image histogram attains a bizarre, unexpected shape from the image data when:
    –Multiple exposure errors _____
    –Very _____ exposure conditions exist

80. For example, if the computer locates S_{MIN} too far to the left because of a large prosthesis, the S_{AVE} of the VOI moves too far left, and the computer may _____ toward a dark image.

81. Digital processing is very robust in correcting for most typical fogging events caused during _____.

82. Most typical localized fog patterns do not alter the shape of the acquired image histogram enough to throw off _____ identification.

83. However, "____-fogging" of a CR cassette affects primarily the lighter portions of the image, adding a large number of light gray pixels at the left of the histogram, and leaving no "blank" white pixels present. This skews the location of S_{MIN} and S_{AVE}, and can remain uncorrected.

84. If a CR plate has been "fogged" by either background or scatter radiation prior to using it for a radiographic exposure, digital processing is NOT generally able to _____ for the effects of pre-fogging the plate.

85. DR detector plates are automatically _____ between exposures, and are not vulnerable to "pre-fogging"—a "fogged" appearing image is very rare for DR.

86. Various histogram analysis and _____ errors can result in an image that is too light, too dark, with excessive contrast or with excessive gray scale.

87. Most digital processing errors are _____ to the original radiographic technique used.

Chapter 6

RESCALING (PROCESSING) THE DIGITAL RADIOGRAPH

1. Digitization results in a _____ number of gray levels (pixel values) assigned to "bins" or computer files.

2. This range, far beyond the discernment of the human eye, allows for _____ up and down within the dynamic range.

3. A set of numerical data can be _____ in all sorts of ways, allowing levelling and windowing.

4. Anything that alters the _____ of the histogram represents a change in contrast or gray scale. Two examples include using exponential functions (see textbook) and numerical rounding.

5. Applying an exponential function (formula), for example, can result in a set of pixel values that increases and decreases in increments of 4 rather than in increments of 2. The final image will be displayed with increased _____.

6. Depending on the degree to which incoming pixel values are rounded up or down, they can be made to fit a pre-set _____ of S values.

7. More severe rounding results in _____ values.

8. In the histogram, more severe rounding results in fewer vertical _____, representing fewer pixel values present in the image.

9. In the displayed image, this is _____ gray scale.

10. The computer CAN align the average _____ of the image. This is leveling.

Rescaling (Processing) the Digital Radiograph 39

11. By aligning the high and low points of the S and Q ranges, the computer CAN roughly _____ the gray scale, thus the contrast, of the image. This can be done by using more severe rounding of pixel values.

12. This is _____.

13. What CANNOT be done by the computer is to force the specific shape of the histograms to match by altering the pixel _____ in each bin.

14. This would require changing _____ pixels across the image hold a particular initial value—We can change pixel values, not pixel counts.

"Normalizing" the Image

15. *Rescaling* is re-mapping the brightness and gray scale of the digital image so that it appears like a "_____" or conventional radiograph.

16. A "raw" digital image directly from the image receptor appears "washed-out," with extremely low _____.

17. _____ corrects the brightness, and partially corrects the gray scale for each image.

18. The final displayed image nearly always has ideal brightness and gray scale, _____ of the technique used on initial exposure.

Q Values and the Permanent LUT (Look-Up Table)

19. Rescaling can be done electronically or with software. _____ has several advantages and is the more common method.

20. The KEY to rescaling is to algebraically assign the _____ labels to incoming data regardless of what the data actually is.

21. A permanent look-up table of ___ values is stored in the computer.

22. The Q values in this permanent look-up table represent the "ideal" _____ for the anatomical procedure.

23. For the *acquired* histogram, "bins" of data from the acquired image to be used for rescaling are designated as ___ values.

24. The "____" of data between S_MIN and S_MAX are designated as S2, S3, S4 and so on up to S_MAX.

25. For the *acquired* histogram, the full range of acquired image _____ is used, ranging from S_MIN and S_MAX.

26. For *rescaling* of the image, to align the acquired image data with the output scale of this permanent LUT (the "ideal" histogram), the range of S values from incoming histogram must _____ the number of Q values in the table.

27. To rescale the image, a computer algorithm remaps incoming S values to ___ values.

28. Re-mapping the image means that regardless of the specific input values, the output values are always the _____.

29. It is this data set (the Q values) that are later fed into the anatomical LUT for _____ processing.

30. Gradation processing will refine the image according to the specific _____ procedure.

31. Rescaling always corrects for brightness because the histogram of the S values is always re-_____ to the Q value range.

32. Physicists refer to "for _____" values of pixels that have undergone preprocessing corrections, but *have not yet been rescaled,* as Q values.

33. Physicists refer to *rescaled* pixel values as ____ values.

34. Physicists define Q_P values as the finalized "for _____" pixel values after all postprocessing operations are complete. These will be displayed at the monitor.

35. To minimize confusion, we will use "S" values for _____ data from the acquired histogram.

36. To minimize confusion, we will use "Q" Values for all _____ values.

Chapter 7

DEFAULT POSTPROCESSING I: GRADATION PROCESSING

Digital Processing domains

1. List the three general approaches to sorting any field-of-view:
   By _____
   By _____
   By _____
   (See car shopping example in textbook.)

2. The same three methods apply to sorting an image for digital processing. The method chosen by the manufacturer depends on which one is most _____ for a particular outcome.

3. In the SPATIAL Domain, pixels are sorted by their _____.

4. In the INTENSITY Domain, pixels are sorted by their pixel _____ (gray levels).

5. In the FREQUENCY Domain, _____ (details) are sorted by their size.

6. In the Spatial Domain, pixels are acted upon according to their location within the image _____.

7. In the Intensity Domain, pixels are operated upon based on their gray levels. At the display monitor, the pixel value determines amount of _____ applied.

8. This, in turn, determines the _____ level displayed for the pixel.

9. These operations are all controlled by _____ *transformation formulas*.

10. In the Frequency Domain, large objects are _____-frequency structures (see Chap. 8).

11. In the Frequency Domain, small objects are _____-frequency structures (see Chap. 8).

12. Sorting an image by pixel *location* results in a _____.

13. Sorting an image by pixel *intensity* (brightness) results in a _____.

14. Sorting an image by *object* _____ results in a frequency distribution.

15. The *histogram* plots the _____ of pixels against each pixel value.

16. The frequency distribution plots the number of _____ or details against their size.

17. The frequency distribution is similar to a histogram, but with _____ vertical bars (dozens rather than hundreds).

18. While the image is separated into the intensity domain (histogram), specific _____ can be targeted to be altered.

19. Each density is stored in a separate computer _____.

20. While the image is separated into the frequency domain, specific _____ of objects or details can be targeted for enhancement or suppression.

21. Each size of object is stored in a _____ computer file.

22. Every image begins and ends in the _____ domain.

23. As pixels are sorted by their intensity, transitioning the image into the intensity domain, or as objects are sorted by their size, transitioning the image into the frequency domain, the computer keeps track of the _____ locations they occupied, so they can be placed back after intensity or frequency processing is completed.

Default Postprocessing I: Gradation Processing 43

24. A *kernel* is a _____ that is passed over the original pixels of the image, executing some mathematical function on them.

25. Applied to re-set the value in each pixel, row by row, this is a _____-processing operation.

26. As a kernel moves left-to-right across a row of the image matrix, each _____ value will be subtracted from, added tom, multiplied by, or divided by the factors in the *bottom row* of the kernel.

27. As the kernel then indexes down, the middle values in the _____ will be applied to each pixel in the same matrix row, then the top values will be applied.

28. All nine cells of the kernel will eventually sweep over each pixel in the _____ matrix.

29. After all rows of the image matrix have been swept over horizontally by rows, the same operations are repeated vertically by _____.

30. By using different values or _____ in the cells of the kernel, all kinds of changes can be made to the image, such as increasing or decreasing overall contrast.

31. Spatial Domain Operations can be further subdivided into:
    1. _____ Processing Operations
    2. _____ Processing Operations
    3. _____ Processing Operations

32. Point Processing Operations perform a specific algorithm on _____ pixel in sequence, pixel by pixel (point by point). Example: subtraction.

33. Area Processing Operations execute a function on a local _____ of pixels or subsection of the image. Example: Zoom (magnification).

34. Global Operations carry out a massive spatial function across the _____ area of the image. Examples: Rotate, invert, or translate the image.

35. *Intensity domain operations* include histogram construction & _____, gradation processing (this chapter), and _____.

36. These operations affect all pixels holding a particular _____, regardless of their location in the matrix.

37. *Frequency operations* include edge _____, smoothing, and background suppression.

38. These operations target a specific size of _____ for modification, for example, edge enhancement enhances only the _____ contrast of fine details, without changing overall image contrast.

Gradation Processing

39. The purpose of Gradation Processing is to refine the contrast according to the _____.

40. Gradation: "A gradual passing from one tint or shade to another" = _____ _____.

41. Gradient: "The rate of change in an ascending or descending _____; the steepness of a slope.

42. Gradation or gradient processing is named after the gradient curve of an image. The left-to-right position of the curve indicates resulting image brightness, while the steepness of the curve represents resulting image _____.

43. Every image is subjected to gradient processing as part of _____ processing.

44. Windowing is actually a _____ of gradient processing.

45. Window level controls brightness, the left-to-right _____ of the curve.

46. Window width controls contrast, the _____ of the curve.

47. The anatomical LUT (Look-Up Table) to be applied is determined when the operator selects the anatomical procedure at the _____.

48. A permanent anatomical _____ is stored by the computer for each procedure.

49. For Gradation Processing, the _____ data set is fed into the anatomical LUT.

50. The anatomical LUT customizes the gray scale and brightness according to the specific _____ to be demonstrated.

51. Look-Up Tables really are tables, (not _____).

52. Graphs used to represent LUTs are for _____ benefit in understanding them.

53. The computer deals in _____, not in graphs.

54. The conversion of input values to output values is generated by a _____ or algorithm that can be represented as a *function curve* on a graph.

55. A graph representing a typical LUT plots the input pixel values along the bottom axis, and the converted output pixel values, reflected off the _____ curve, on the vertical (abscissa).

56. The actual look-up table is simply a _____ of the input values and then the output values resulting from these mathematical operations.

57. All gradation processing takes place in the _____ domain.

58. The types of formulas used for gradation processing are referred to as intensity _____.

59. These are the same formulas applied whenever the radiographer _____ the image after it is initially displayed.

60. The type (shape) of curve used by each manufacturer represents the _____ function (formula) applied to set up the anatomical LUT.

61. Different parameters entered into the formulas change the position or slope of the _____.

62. When windowing the formulas and parameters used first set up the LUT, then output is simply _____ out from the LUT as input is fed into it.

63. (For rescaling, an _____-generated permanent LUT was used: Input values were assigned to pre-set labels and output was simply read out from the LUT.)

64. Gradient Processing is used, first, during _____ processing when anatomical LUTs are applied, and second, any time the displayed image is _____ by the operator.

Data Clipping

65. If either the dynamic range or the bit depth of a digital processing system is too _____, it is possible for data clipping to occur when either brightness or contrast are adjusted (leveling or windowing).

66. The dynamic range of the software, supported by the _____ of the computer hardware, must extend sufficiently above and below typical input values to allow for all probable adjustments to the image.

67. If the dynamic range is too short, the darkest pixel values can be truncated (cut off) from the image either by increasing window _____ or by increasing _____.

68. In either case, data is _____ from the displayed image, which may compromise proper diagnosis.

Dynamic Range Compression

69. Since the bit depth of a computer far exceeds the range of human vision, memory _____ space can be saved by not using the entire bit depth of the system.

70. Enough dynamic range must remain to still allow the image to be _____ or _____ (leveled).

71. Mathematically, DRC finds the mid-point of the gray scale curve, then progressively _____ pixel values above this point, and progressively _____ pixel values below it.

72. Applied to a degree visibly affecting the image, this results in tissue _____, a cutting off of the darkest and lightest densities.

73. Visible DRC is also known as "tissue equalization" or "_____ equalization."

Default Postprocessing I: Gradation Processing 47

74. With conventional radiography, when soft tissue techniques were used to demonstrate soft tissue areas, bones were then depicted too _____.

75. By truncating the gray scale curve, DRC brings extremely light densities up to a darker level, and extremely dark areas are made lighter. This is an even better result (than conventional soft-tissue technique), since _____ are also still demonstrated well.

76. DRC _____ conventional "soft-tissue technique."

77. Conventional soft tissue technique consisted of reducing the kVp by 20% with no compensation in mAs, to both reduce penetration and _____ the image overall.

78. Rescaling is designed to _____ produce the same overall brightness and contrast.

79. Therefore, if conventional soft tissue technique is used, digital processing will simply _____ and cancel it out.

80. Tissue equalization effects of DRC: Since the darkest areas (lung fields below) are lightened, while the lightest areas (mediastinum below) are darkened, the resulting densities range from _____ _____ to _____ _____.

81. Dynamic Range Compression is better described as "gray scale _____.

82. DRC is a _____ off of the extreme ends of the gray scale.

83. Using DRC for gray scale truncation can be very confusing: Elimination of darkest and lightest densities in gray scale range results in a _____-looking image!

84. This seems to contradict conventional _____ of gray scale which results in increased contrast.

85. Lengthening gray scale by increasing kVp makes the image look "grayer" because there are _____ shades of gray present.

86. DRC makes the image look "grayer" because the lightest and darkest shades are now _____!

87. Conventional shortening of gray scale (left) may be thought of as "squeezing" the range of densities that still extends from _____ to _____.

88. DRC actually _____ the whites and blacks out of the gray scale.

Chapter 8

DEFAULT POSTPROCESSING II: DETAIL PROCESSING

1. Detail processing is characterized by its ability to treat fine details as a _____ component of the image, without changing the overall brightness or contrast of the image as a whole.

2. Detail processing decouples _____ contrast from global contrast.

3. Detail processing can be performed either in the _____ domain, using kernels, or in the frequency domain, using Fourier analysis.

Understanding the Frequency Domain

4. From Chapter 3, recall that an "exposure trace diagram" somewhat resembles a _____ moving up and down.

5. Either by mathematical averaging, or by adding the effects of penumbral blur, this squared graph becomes _____ to appear like a sine wave.

6. A _____ of these sign waves (modulation transfer function) is created when a resolution template is exposed.

7. On a display monitor, a single _____ of pixels can be sampled such that the values of the pixels across its length form a sine-wave graph.

8. Compared to alternating black and white pixels, a row of alternating gray and white pixels results in a graph with waves having less _____ or height.

9. On this graph, the _____ is representative of the size (width) of the pixels.

10. On a display monitor, if an *entire row* of pixels from the left edge to the right edge of the screen consists of 600 pixels, this row has a _____ of 300 Hertz.

11. (Each cycle is made of __ pulses or __ pixels.)

12. The frequency of a row of hardware pixels on a monitor depends on the _____ (_____) of the pixels.

13. An object and a space within the image also have a frequency related to the number of pixels they _____ in each row.

14. If 2 objects and spaces can just fit across the display screen, they have a lateral frequency of __ Hertz.

15. Five objects and spaces across the display screen have a lateral frequency of 5 _____.

16. Five-Hertz objects must be _____ than 2-Hertz objects to "fit" across the screen.

17. Smaller objects maker shorter waves, and are considered _____-frequency objects because a high number of them "fit" across the screen.

18. Gray level (brightness or density) of each object becomes the amplitude (_____) of the waves.

19. Size of objects (number of pixels occupied by each object) becomes the wavelength (_____) of each wave (i.e., also its frequency).

20. A row of pixel values is represented by a complex sine-wave pattern. Fourier transformation can break this into the individual _____ that make it up.

21. When two water waves of differing wavelengths overlap, they form a _____ wave.

22. A complex wave is the _____ of various waves with different frequencies.

23. Each frequency layer is stored by the computer as a separate _____ or image.

Default Postprocessing II: Detail Processing

24. Each image layer is composed only of details (pixel pairs) with a certain _____.

Frequency Detail Processing

25. In the digital image, the highest frequency layers depict only the _____ details.

26. The lowest frequency layers depict only the largest _____.

27. The dark "background" density is _____ from the high-frequency layers, because it is treated as a large "structure" with very low-frequency.

28. *Multiscale processing* decomposes the original image into 8 or more frequency _____, targeting specific layers for detail processing operations, then recomposing the image.

29. The original image is split into a high-frequency and a low-frequency component, then the ____-frequency layer is split again and again in series.

30. While separated, different operations (such as gradation processing) can be executed on any _____ image layer.

31. By choosing which frequency to boost, we can choose which _____ of structures in the image to enhance.

32. The altered layer can then be placed back into the _____ for reconstruction by inverse Fourier transformation.

33. The _____ of details in only that layer (of only that size) is enhanced relative to other layers.

34. After these operations are completed, *inverse Fourier transformation* _____ the image by adding the component waves back together.

35. In the final image displayed on the monitor, the voltage or amperage applied to each row of pixels is controlled by the highs and lows of the complex waveform, thus varying the _____ level of each pixel displayed.

36. Any image layer can be entirely _____ upon reconstructing the image.

37. _____-pass Filtering is named after the frequency layers it "passes through" or leaves in the image.

38. Low-Pass Filtering is widely used for _____ dexel drop-out or default noise reduction for electronic (periodic) mottle.

39. Since these forms of noise have a consistent size, they tend to be concentrated in ____ frequency layer.

40. Applied as a postprocessing feature at the console, low-pass filtering is generically known as _____, although different manufacturers use different names.

41. The trade-off for smoothing (low-pass filtering) is a _____ of some finer details that may be of diagnostic value, along with slightly blurrier edges.

42. Elimination of noise from the image generally requires that we accept the loss of some _____ detail along with it.

43. High-pass filtering targets one or more mid- to low-frequency layers to be _____.

44. *Background suppression* refers to elimination of the very _____ frequencies.

45. Applied as a postprocessing feature at the console, high-pass filtering is most commonly known as _____ _____, (although different manufacturers use different names)

46. The result of edge enhancement is that _____ details and fine edges stand out better against the surrounding larger anatomy.

47. The trade-off for edge enhancement is a slightly more _____ image.

48. Over-application of edge enhancement can result in a loss of _____.

49. Some manufacturers _____ EE with other processing steps under various proprietary names.

50. Any image _____ can be boosted, suppressed, removed, or subjected to gradient processing, noise reduction, or other treatments.

Default Postprocessing II: Detail Processing   53

51. Every image begins and ends in the _____ domain.

52. The computer keeps track of the matrix _____ different objects occupied, so they can be placed back after frequency processing is completed.

53. The use of kernels for detail processing is a *spatial* operation. In this case, ___ transition into another domain is necessary.

Spatial Detail Processing: Kernels as a Form of Band-Pass Processing

54. Kernels can perform spatial detail processing, when simple _____ factors are placed in its cells.

55. The _____ of the kernel's matrix determines a transition frequency between enhancement and suppression.

56. Small details with a frequency above this transition point are _____.

57. Large structures with a frequency below this point are _____.

58. This is equivalent to _____-pass processing.

59. Kernel operations pass a smaller "____-_____" of core values over each pixel row by row, then column by column, assigning new pixel values by *interpolation*.

60. Each pixel value is _____ by the "core" values in the kernel, (resulting in fractions).

61. These fractional values are then _____ to assign a new value to the centered pixel.

62. The location of any kernel over the matrix is defined by which pixel its _____ cell is centered over.

63. A center cell can be identified only for _____-dimension kernels.

64. A given pixel will be multiplied by _____ cell in the kernel in series as it passes over row by row.

65. The entire process is then repeated _____ column by column (see Chapter 7 for further clarification).

66. The effect (smoothing, edge enhancement, or background suppression) depends on the _____ between the multiplying factors in the kernel.

67. Every detail processing effect that can be achieved in the _____ domain can also be achieved in the spatial domain using kernel operations.

68. Kernels can even be used to increase or decrease _____ (global) contrast, although gradation processing is more widely used for this purpose.

69. The effects of band-pass _____ can also be achieved.

70. The size of structures to eliminate can be targeted: The larger the kernel (more cells), the _____ the structures suppressed.

71. Too _____ a kernel can remove important details; too large a kernel may be ineffective.

72. *"Unsharp" Mask Filtering* is a method of edge enhancement. In step #1. A kernel is used to separate the _____, gross structures into a separate image layer.

73. In step #2, a _____ of the "unsharp" mask is created by image reversal.

74. In step #3, this positive _____ is effectively superimposed over the original image.

75. This causes the positive and negative pixel values to _____ each other out to subtract gross structures present on both images.

76. The resulting image shows _____ details better. This is a form of low-pass filtering.

Preparation for Display

77. Many manufacturers perform additional gradation processing and noise reduction prior to display: To avoid inadvertent "cropping of the image," the number of pixels in the _____ of the PACS stored image must match the number of pixels available on the display monitor.

78. The dynamic range of the PACS stored image must also _____ with the bit depth of the display monitor to allow a full range of windowing without data clipping.

79. Algorithms to align these parameters are usually included within the _____ monitor itself.

Chapter 9

MANIPULATING THE DIGITAL IMAGE: OPERATOR ADJUSTMENTS

1. All *operator adjustments* are considered _____ as we have defined it.

2. These are changes made at the console after _____ processing is completed and the initial image is _____.

3. Examples include leveling and _____, applying alternate algorithms, and applying special features such as smoothing, edge enhancement, background suppression, image stitching for scoliosis, grid line suppression and processing suites used by different manufacturers.

Processing Algorithms

4. When a radiographic procedure is selected at the console, a digital _____ program tailored to that anatomy is being selected, that includes:

    1. The reference _____ for analysis
    2. The "permanent" LUT for _____
    3. The anatomical _____ for default gradation processing
    4. Default _____ processing features for the anatomy

5. One way to adjust the contrast and brightness characteristics of an image is to re-process it under a _____ pre-set anatomical algorithm.

6. For most systems, when you touch the histogram graph displayed at the console, a _____ of body parts or procedures will appear to select from for re-processing.

7. However, use of alternate algorithms should be the _____, not the rule.

8. Since most default processing settings result in ideal image quality, the radiographer should have supervisor or radiologist _____ to use alternate algorithms.

9. However, if an image re-processed under a different algorithm is saved into the PACS, the original data set is permanently _____.

10. This _____ the radiologist's ability to fully window the image.

11. The image is also stored under a changed DICOM header as a _____ procedure, complicating record-keeping and possibly causing legal problems.

12. A workable compromise is to make a _____, re-process the copy under the new algorithm with annotation of the change added to it, then save it to the PACS.

13. Departments should have clear _____ for saving altered images into the PACS.

Windowing

14. Brightness and contrast can be _____ at the console as the image is being viewed.

15. Strictly speaking, as used in CT, *window level* refers to how _____ the image is.

16. "Leveling": _____ window level makes the image darker.

17. However, when window level is raised, the range of the gray scale is _____.

18. Window width can also be changed without changing the _____ density.

19. Strictly speaking, as used in CT, *window width* refers to how long the _____ _____ is.

20. "Windowing": Increasing window width creates _____ gray scale.

58 Student Workbook for Digital Radiography in Practice

21. In CR, DR and DF systems, the user-friendly terms brightness and contrast are commonly used: Increasing brightness is _____ to increasing window level.

22. Increasing contrast is opposite to _____ window width.

23. Window level ____ be changed without changing window width. Window width ____ be changed without altering window level.

24. As discussed in Chapter 3, an image can be made darker or lighter without altering _____.

25. As discussed in Chapter 3, contrast or gray scale can also be changed without altering the average (overall) _____.

26. When leveling and windowing are applied to an image and then it is saved into the PAC system, the range of windowing available to the radiologist is always _____.

27. The _____ image data should always be preserved for the radiologist.

28. If altered images are saved into the PACS, they should be saved as separate _____.

Postprocessing Features

29. Smoothing algorithms remove some of the smallest details (highest _____ layers) from the image.

30. The results of smoothing include:

    1. Edges of bony structures appear "_____" due to reduction in local contrast.
    2. _____ is reduced by mathematical interpolation.
    3. Dead or stuck dexels are _____ by mathematical interpolation.

31. All manufacturers apply _____ in some form, although they may use different proprietary names.

32. An important *trade-off* for smoothing is some loss of image _____.

33. For an image already presenting low overall contrast, smoothing may lead to a loss of diagnostic _____, because smoothing ADDS local contrast reduction to the previous loss of overall contrast.

34. Local contrast can be changed without affecting _____ contrast—This is what smoothing and edge enhancement do.

35. BUT, changing overall contrast DOES affect local contrast because _____ details are included.

36. Smoothing is recommended to suppress moderate amounts of _____ in the image.

37. _____ mottle represents substantial underexposure which may include a loss of small details.

38. Smoothing algorithms will not recover lost information due to severe _____.

39. Radiographs presenting severe mottle from underexposure should be _____.

40. Edge Enhancement brings out _____ details against larger background structures.

41. Edge enhancement increases local contrast: Small pathological changes, such as a "hairline" fracture, may become more _____.

42. An important *trade-off* for edge enhancement is that it increases visibility of image _____ including mottle, which may have been initially present but not at a bothersome visible level, and now is.

43. This is especially true if the original image already possessed high _____.

44. For a very high-contrast image, edge enhancement may cause artifacts including the _____ effect.

45. In this effect, at the boundary between two anatomical structures, the darker density side is ____-darkened while the lighter side is lightened even more.

46. Different terms are used by different manufacturers. For example: GE's "look" feature includes "normal, hard and soft" settings: The "hard look" engages _____. The "soft look" engages _____ algorithms.

47. Clinical cases have shown that the _____ amount of edge enhancement can be excessive enough to obscure a hairline fracture in a bone-dense area.

48. It is possible to _____-apply edge enhancement or smoothing, especially if the original image has very high or very low initial contrast, respectively.

49. Both smoothing and edge enhancement should be used with discretion. Always _____ results with the original image.

50. Default settings for edge enhancement and smoothing in the system can be _____ by the quality control technologist in password-protected menus, in consultation with radiologists.

51. *Background suppression* algorithms reduce the contrast only of _____ mid-frequency and low-frequency structures.

52. The effect is very similar to edge enhancement, but it can be more effective for _____ situations like muscular fat pad overlapping bone marrow details.

53. Software programs can target specific _____ of the image for brightness correction (eliminating the need for compensating filters for many procedures).

54. *Dark masking* reverses blank areas around the image to a _____ border.

55. Dark masking reduces extraneous glare, improving apparent _____, and is always recommended.

56. Dark masking should _____ be used to "re-collimate" an image taken with too large an exposure field.

57. Radiologists are legally responsible for ____ diagnostic information on the initial radiograph, even if it is unrelated to the purpose for which it was ordered.

58. *Image reversal,* sometimes called "black bone" reverses image to "_____-on-_____" (_____ background).

Manipulating the Digital Image: Operator Adjustments 61

59. All pixel _____ are reversed, darkest to lightest, second-darkest to second-lightest, and so on.

60. Image reversal produces no _____ information in the image, but can make some details subjectively more apparent.

61. *Image stitching* is used for scoliosis series. Three CR plates can be quickly exposed over the cervical, thoracic, and lumbar areas while the patient remains in position. These exposures _____ each other a few centimeters.

62. Using a special alignment grid, image stitching software can accurately align the three images to form a _____ body-length image.

63. DR has the same capability, but uses a _____ detector and only requires 2 exposures.

64. *Dual energy subtraction* is capable of separating the digital image into a tissue only image and a bone only image. These images aid diagnosis by _____ obstructing anatomy.

65. In order to produce separate soft tissue and bone images, a high-energy image and a low energy image must first be obtained, having very different _____ characteristics.

66. Two methods are available for obtaining these two images: In the first method, a double-exposure is made at two different _____ settings. About 200 milliseconds (1/5 sec) is required between exposures for switching the kVp, (allowing possible motion).

67. In the second method, a single exposure is made of a special receptor system that includes a _____ placed between two or more imaging plates.

68. For the filter method, a cassette with two or three image receptor plates is used. The first plate records a low-energy beam. A thick filter hardens the x-ray beam reaching the 2nd plate, so the average _____ of the x-rays is much higher.

69. At higher kVp levels, photoelectric interactions drop more precipitously for soft tissue than for bone so the contrast for soft tissues changes _____ dramatically. This provides a measurement the computer can use to identify soft tissues in order to separate them from bones in the output image:

70. Comparing these two exposures, the computer identifies soft tissue areas as those where photoelectric absorption _____ for the high-energy image.

71. The computer then subtracts the remaining _____ areas from the identified soft tissue areas.

72. *Grid lines* can be characterized as a low-frequency phenomenon which occurs in a _____ axis in the image (vertically).

73. *Grid line suppression* software allows the computer to identify them and subtract them from the image, by leaving out the corresponding _____ layer upon reconstructing the image (band-pass filtering).

74. ANY type of artifacts that have _____ and consistent characteristics (such as tomographic streaks) can be identified by computer software for elimination.

Chapter 10

MONITORING AND CONTROLLING EXPOSURE

Digital Speed Class

1. The speed of any imaging system expresses its _____ to radiation.

2. Historically, speed was always _____ related to the amount of exposure required to produce an adequate signal at the image receptor

    Speed = $\dfrac{1}{\text{Exposure Required}}$

3. If twice the exposure required = _____ the speed.

4. For film-based radiography, a standard speed value of ____ was defined as requiring an exposure of 20 microgray to produce a medium gray density.

5. A 50-speed film was half as "fast," and required _____ the exposure to achieve the same density.

6. By comparison, the inherent speed of a typical CR phosphor plate is about ____.

7. However, for digital systems, the inherent speed of the IR is important only at the image acquisition stage, and is only half the story—The speed of the system as a whole is determined by the digital _____ used.

8. Operating speed can be _____ without any physical change to the IR.

9. Since the speed at which a digital system operates can be selected, it is referred to as speed _____ rather than just "speed."

10. The 100 speed class assumes an average exposure of ____ μGy will penetrate through to the image receptor. A 200 speed class assumes 10 μGy, and a 400 speed class assumes 5 μGy.

11. Immediately before the advent of digital imaging systems, the most commonly used film/screen combinations in radiography had a speed of _____.

12. Early CR readers (processors) were typically installed to operate at a speed class of _____.

13. This was a step _____ for patient dose.

14. Now, nearly all CR and DR units can be operated at a speed class of _____-_____, without the appearance of mottle.

15. Doing so saves patient _____ to harmful radiation.

A Brief History of Exposure Indicators

16. For digital systems, since the image has always been manipulated by the computer, neither its brightness nor its contrast can be attributed entirely to the original radiographic _____ used by the radiographer.

17. In fact, digital images taken at increased technique sometimes turn out _____ in appearance.

18. This means that there is no immediate, obvious feedback (reinforcement) to the radiographer when _____ technique has been used for an exposure.

19. Although, gross underexposure may be indicated by the appearance of _____.

20. Manufacturers developed numerical exposure _____ to provide feedback to the radiographer on the exposure level to the image receptor.

21. Exposure indicators are *not* related to the brightness level of the image _____.

22. Nor are exposure indicators a direct measurement of actual exposure to the _____.

Monitoring and Controlling Exposure

23. For most manufacturers, the exposure indicator (EI) is not an actual exposure reading taken at the image receptor, but is _____ by the computer from reading the midway point (between S_{MIN} and S_{MAX}) on the same image histogram generated for processing.

24. From this average, each manufacturer provides a _____ exposure indicator (EI_T) that represents the "ideal" amount of x-ray exposure at the IR.

25. The EI_T is not inherent to the system. Rather, the desired speed class for different procedures is determined by management, then the appropriate EI_T for that _____ _____ is derived.

26. General types of scales used for exposure indicators include logarithmic scales, proportional scales, and inversely proportional scales. Different _____ approaches are used by different manufacturers. Standardization was severely needed!

The Deviation Index: Acceptable Parameters for Exposure

27. In 2009, the American Association of Medical Physicists (AAMP) recommended a standardized _____ _____ (DI) for use between all manufacturers.

28. The DI should be "prominently _____" immediately after every exposure.

29. The standardized DI is based on actual exposure to the image _____ measured in microgray.

30. The DI is to be permanently stored as part of the DICOM _____ (metadata) for each image in the PACS.

31. Anything which can lead to histogram analysis errors can cause the exposure indicator to be _____.

32. List three examples:

33. A universal formula is used to _____ the DI.

34. Action _____ are published by the AAPM (American Association of Physicists in Medicine).

35. "The index changes by +1.0 for each +___% (increase in exposure), and by –1.0 for each –___% change," but these are multiplicative, not additive.

36. Each step _____ the previous amount (not the original amount) by 1.259 when increasing, by 0.794 when decreasing.

37. Indicators of +__ or –__ are roughly equivalent to a factor of 2 (double, or one-half, ideal exposure).

38. "The index changes by +1.0 for each +25% (increase in exposure), and by –1.0 for each –20% change." These percentage changes are actually _____ changes:

39. 125% of the original exposure is ____ as a ratio. 80% (minus 20%) exposure is _____ as a ratio. Inverted ratios are proportionate changes.

40. Percentages can be tricky, it is easier to use _____ to understand this math.

41. For example: Double a number is a 100% increase. One-half a number is a 50% decrease, yet both are changed by a ratio of __.

42. An exposure less than 80% of the EI$_T$ should _____ be repeated unless a radiologist finds the level of mottle in the image unacceptable.

43. Only exposures less than ____% of the EI$_T$ is EI$_T$ should be assumed to be repeatable.

44. No _____ digital image should be repeated, no matter the EI$_T$, unless saturation has occurred!

45. Like filled buckets spilling water over into each other, electrical charge can overwhelm the capacity of the dexels to store it, _____ across an area of the detector plate. This is saturation.

46. With _____ read-outs at maximum value, there ceases to be any distinction between pixels, i.e., no image to process.

47. The reason the Deviation Index table urges "no repeat" for images that are simply too dark is because these are caused by failures in digital processing and can generally be _____ through additional windowing.

Monitoring and Controlling Exposure   67

48. True saturation, on the other hand, is an _____ phenomenon that occurs at the detector, not during digital processing. Therefore, it cannot be corrected by _____.

49. Extreme over-exposure can overwhelm the digital _____ system, causing a loss of data that results in a flat black appearance of the over- exposed portion of the image.

50. This is not "fog," but a _____ of data.

51. If any details at all can be made out in the dark portion of the image, it is _____ or _____ but NOT saturation.

52. True saturation presents a flat black area with absolutely ___ details present.

53. It takes at least ___ to ___ times the normal exposure to reach saturation. For several manufacturers, it takes even more. This corresponds to an exposure index number of 3000 for the CareStream (Kodak) system, or an S number of 25 for Fuji.

54. So, saturation is rare, and in most instances of overexposure the computer system is able to perfectly _____ such that the final image has good quality.

Limitations of the DI

The deviation index is:

55. One indicator, not ___ indicator, of image quality.

56. An indicator, not a _____, of patient exposure.

57. Taken from data at the image _____, (not at the patient's surface or within the patient), the DI is a "guide to exposure intended to indicate the acceptability of signal-to-noise ratio conditions."

A Note on "Controlling" Factors

58. Since the advent of digital imaging, only one of the five image qualities (shape distortion) can still be attributed to the "controlling _____ factors" traditionally taught.

59. These old "controlling factors" still apply to the latent image carried by the remnant beam to the IR, but not to the final _____ digital image.

Chapter 11

DIGITAL IMAGE ACQUISITION

1. In the digital age, there are two general types of x-ray machines:
    1. _____
    2. _____

2. DR is further broken down into:
    1. _____-conversion DR units
    2. _____-conversion DR units

3. In CR (Computed Radiography), the image receptor has no direct _____ to the processor—the cassette must be physically carried to the CR reader

4. CR was first introduced as "_____-less" radiography.

5. DR (Digital Radiography) doesn't require the image receptor to be _____ to a processor separate from the exposure unit.

6. The IR is directly connected, electrically or electromagnetically (by _____ waves), to the processor.

7. DR was first introduced as "_____-less" radiography (although *mobile* units now use a "cassette."

8. The main image-capture component of all DR detectors is the active matrix _____ (AMA), a flat panel consisting of thousands of individual detector elements referred to as dexels or dels.

9. Typical size for modern detector elements (dexels) is about 100 microns, 1/____th millimeter or about 1/____th the size of a pinhead.

10. This size of dexels is just at the _____ of human vision at normal reading distance.

11. It results in an image that appears _____ at a distance, as sharp as the human eye can detect.

12. These thin AMAs led to _____-panel technology.

13. For Direct-Conversion DR, the AMA panel converts energy of remnant x-ray beam directly into _____ charges that can be "read out" to the computer.

14. For Indirect-Conversion DR, a phosphorescent "screen" is laid over the _____. This screen converts x-rays into _____, which then strikes the AMA panel below.

15. For Direct-Conversion DR, the detection surface of each dexel is made of amorphous _____.

16. Selenium is more sensitive to high-energy _____.

17. For Indirect-Conversion DR, the detection surface of each dexel made of amorphous _____.

18. Silicon is more sensitive to low-energy _____ from the phosphor plate.

19. *Amorphous* means "without shape," a non-crystalline _____.

Direct-Conversion DR Detectors

20. For DR, a *dexel* (detector element) consists of a semiconductor detection surface about _____ thick, a TFT (thin film transistor) for a "switch," and a microscopic capacitor.

21. The heart of the dexel is the microscopic electronic _____.

22. The capacitor's ability to _____ electric charge makes direct-capture imaging possible.

Digital Image Acquisition 71

23. The amount of charge stored will eventually be represented as the _____ _____ (gray level) for each pixel.

24. In each dexel, the TFT (thin film transistor) acts as a switching _____ to release the built-up electrical charge when the dexel is "read out."

25. On exposure, x-rays or light ionize molecules of selenium or silicon, creating an electron-hole _____.

26. (The "hole" consists of the ionized molecule with a _____ charge).

27. The top electrode attracts freed electrons to drift upward. The dexel electrode below has a _____ charge applied, attracting the positively-charged "holes" to drift downward.

28. "Hole drift" actually consists of electrons from each successive layer below being pulled upward, thus leaving gaps or holes in each successive _____ layer.

29. Positive charge from the lower electrode is _____ in the capacitor.

30. Electrical charge built up on the capacitor is proportional to x-ray _____ received.

31. The array of dexels is criss-crossed by _____ called gate lines and data lines.

32. Gate lines are controlled by the address driver, which controls the _____ in which the dexels are read out.

33. When the *bias* voltage applied to a gate line is changed from –5V to +10V, the _____ "gates" open in sequence and dump their charge into a data line.

34. This surge of charge flows to an amplifier, then to the computer through an _____.

35. The sudden change of voltage from negative to positive effectively "_____ the TFT "gate."

36. A _____ of conductivity is created through the detection layer, allowing charge to flow from the capacitor out the TFT.

37. Charge is "dumped" from each dexel into the _____ line in succession.

38. An electronic amplifier _____ this signal, then passes it through an analog-to-digital converter (ADC) to the computer.

Indirect-Conversion DR Detectors

39. In an indirect conversion system, the entire AMA (active matrix array) is overlaid with a _____ screen (or scintillation layer) made of cesium iodide or gadolinium oxysulfide.

40. The active matrix array (AMA) below is the same as that used for direct-conversion systems, only the dexels use amorphous _____ rather than amorphous selenium.

41. The phosphor screen scintillates or fluoresces when exposed to x-rays, emitting _____ which will strike the AMA of TFT detectors below.

42. Although vertical crystals form light channels that confine lateral dispersion of light somewhat, the final _____ achieved is still not as good as with a Direct Conversion System.

43. In the AMA below, the process within each dexel itself is identical to that for a _____-conversion system:

44. First, _____/hole pairs are created by ionization.

45. Second, positive _____ drifts downward and is stored on a capacitor.

46. (The greater the stored charge, the _____ the pixel will be upon display.)

47. Finally, charges are "_____ out" by the AMA's data lines, amplified, and passed through an ADC to the computer.

Computed Radiography (CR)

48. The CR cassette is designed in most respects to be used just as screen _____ were used for film-based radiography, and has somewhat similar construction.

49. The active phosphor layer is supported by a firm base, usually made of _____.

50. The CR cassette is usually made of aluminum or plastic with a ____-absorbing carbon fiber front.

51. The back panel may include thin sheet of lead foil to reduce _____ radiation.

52. Both front and back panels of the CR cassette are lined with _____ material that minimizes build-up of static electricity and cushions the plate from jolts.

53. Unlike film cassettes, there is no need for the CR cassette to be _____-tight.

54. For most CR systems, the phosphor plate has only one single emulsion surface and must be inserted facing _____ in the cassette.

55. A small slider _____ at one end of the cassette releases the PSP plate for removal from the slot.

56. Within the CR reader, this button is moved _____ to retrieve and reinsert the PSP plate.

57. In the CR phosphor plate, the reflective layer reverses light traveling _____.

58. The anti-halo layer prevents _____ light from reaching the reflective layer.

59. The phosphor layer converts _____ into visible light.

60. The protective layer is a thin coat of _____.

61. An anti-halo layer added below the phosphor layer is a simple _____ filter which prevents the red light used by the laser beam scanning the plate from penetrating through to the reflective layer, while allowing blue light from the phosphor itself to pass through.

62. The photostimulable phosphor (PSP) is one of a small number of barium-fluoro-halide compounds which possess a unique property called stimulated phosphorescence, the ability to _____ a latent image over time, then release it on stimulation.

63. F Centers (Farbzentren = "color centers") are metastable _____ in the pure crystal structure of a barium fluorohalide compound when doped with europium.

64. F centers act like "electronic holes" that can _____ electrons freed from x-ray ionization of the crystal.

65. F Centers actually form a new _____ band around an atom in which an electron can become "trapped," and later released when energy from a laser is added.

66. The (energy of these) electrons trapped in the F centers forms a _____ image stored by the phosphor plate.

67. Only a small _____ of the electrons are trapped.

68. These electrons are freed from their atoms during an exposure when x-rays _____ the atoms.

69. The image can be _____ (read) after several hours—A typical PSP plate retains up to 75% of the original image 8 hours after exposure.

70. In the CR reader (processor), to release the trapped energy, the crystals are excited by scanning them with a helium-neon red _____ beam.

71. This boost in energy enables the electrons to "jump" out of the traps and "fall back into" their atomic _____.

72. Energy lost from these electrons as they fall back into their shells is emitted as blue-violet _____.

73. In stimulated phosphorescence, absorbed energy from the laser beam enables _____ electrons to "jump" out of the F centers and fall back into their atomic shells.

74. The loss of _____ energy as they fall into their shells is emitted as blue-violet light.

75. The PSP plate actually glows also during x-ray exposure. However, this energy is _____.

Digital Image Acquisition

76. During exposure, the phosphor fluoresces when _____ electrons ejected out of their shells immediately fall back into the shells.

77. However, _____ electrons become trapped in F centers.

78. When the PSP plate is later re-stimulated by the laser beam, it phosphoresces, emitting a very dim light that must be captured and _____ by the CR reader to produce an image.

79. The CR reader uses suction cups to remove the exposed phosphor plate from its cassette, then moves it by a series of _____ through the different sections of the processor.

80. Within the CR reader, the _____ *scan direction* is the direction in which the laser beam scans across the plate.

81. The slow scan (subscan) direction is the direction of _____ movement through the reader.

82. DR dexels are _____ and well-defined.

83. By comparison, the CR laser beam is typically in the shape of an 80-micron _____, so the laser spot must overlap pixels that are being recorded as the plate is read.

84. Unlike DR, the location and size of pixels in CR is defined during _____ rather than by the image receptor.

85. The PSP plate has no defined pixels—it contains an _____ image.

86. The maximum size of these CR pixels is defined by the width of the _____ beam.

87. Their location is defined by the sampling _____—how many measurements are taken across each scan line.

88. Fast scan sampling rate sets their _____.

89. Slow scan sampling rate sets their _____.

90. The light channeling guide is a bundle of _____ fibers that pick up emitted light at a different angle than the incident laser beam, and channel it to the photomuliplier tube (PMT) for amplification.

91. Light emitted by the phosphor plate is changed into an electronic signal by the _____ tube (PM tube), then amplified.

92. The PM tube is a _____ plate attached to an electronic amplifier.

93. Photocathode: A layer of material that releases electrons when light strikes it, through the _____ effect.

94. The amplifier section is a series of _____ plates which can be switched back and forth between positive and negative charge to continuously accelerate and multiply the electron stream.

95. The PM tube is sensitive to a different _____ of light (blue-violet) rather than red.

96. This prevents it from picking up reflected red light from the _____ beam.

97. After scanning, the phosphor plate moves in the subscan direction into the _____ section of the processor, where bright white light is used to completely remove any residual image.

98. The "clean" plate is then _____ into its cassette, and the cassette released for retrieval.

99. Properly erased CR phosphor plates can be _____ thousands of times.

100. Each CR cassette has a unique identifying number that can be accessed by a _____ code reader.

101. Each CR cassette has a blocker area where patient information can be temporarily "_____" onto it.

102. CR phosphor plates are approximately ____ times more sensitive than conventional film to scatter and background radiation accumulated during storage prior to use.

Digital Image Acquisition   77

Background and Scatter Radiation

103. Typical background exposures can be up to 0.8 milligray per day, so over a weekend more than 2 milligray is likely to accumulate. It only takes about ___ milligray to produce a "fog density" on the plate.

104. Radiographers should be careful to _____ any cassette prior to use if there is any chance it has been in storage for 2 days or more.

105. The above describes the sensitivity of the CR plate, not the overall _____, to background and scatter radiation without including an image from which the processor can generate a normal histogram to analyze.

106. Digital processing has a remarkable ability to "clean up" fog densities within the image field caused _____ exposure.

107. It is not, however, able to correct fog densities caused prior to exposure during _____.

108. Since "pre-fogging" a CR cassette ensures that the lightest densities in the latent image will be gray rather than white, the *Contrast-Noise Ratio (CNR)* _____ for the incoming data the computer must process.

109. "Pre-fogging" a cassette adds to the _____ total amount of noise the computer must deal with. If the total amount of all forms of noise becomes overwhelming, histogram analysis can be impaired, causing processing errors.

110. Never leave CR cassettes anywhere in the _____ area, even leaning against walls at some distance.

111. In the bin of a mobile x-ray machine, care must be taken to regularly _____ the CR cassettes.

112. For DR detectors, a "flash" electronic exposure is used to _____ any residual charge between exposures, so the effects of background and scatter radiation are eliminated.

Sharpness of Digital Systems

113. In a CR reader, the only way to increase the sampling frequency, (the number of samples taken per line), is to reduce the _____ between samples.

114. For DR systems, this image sampling frequency depends only upon the dexel pitch, defined as the distance from the _____ of one dexel to the center of an adjacent dexel.

115. Pixel pitch is approximately equal to pixel _____.

116. Dexel pitch is approximately equal to dexel _____.

117. The smaller the dexel or pixel size, the _____ the spatial resolution.

118. (Technically, for DR detectors, the dexel pitch includes any _____ between dexels).

119. The simplest definition for an image detail is the "edge" between _____ pixels with different values (e.g., white and black).

120. Therefore, it takes a minimum of two pixels (with different values) to make a _____.

121. This means that the number of resolvable details is _____ the number of available pixels.

122. To measure sharpness, we use the unit of spatial _____: Line-pairs per millimeter (_____).

123. The maximum spatial resolution is expressed as:

$$SF = \frac{1}{2P}$$

–where P is the _____ or _____ size
–hardware dexels for DR or
–scanned pixels for CR

124. What is the spatial resolution for an imaging system with a dexel pitch of 0.04 mm?

There are several different types of matrices:

125. The _____ matrix of dexels in a DR detector

126. The _____ image matrix created by a CR reader that is sampling a PSP plate

127. The hardware matrix array of _____ pixels (dots) in a display monitor

128. The _____ matrix of the displayed image itself

129. KEY POINT: The size of the matrix and the field-of-view can affect sharpness only if they alter the size of the actual _____ or _____.

130. KEY POINT: For any hardware matrix, the size of the dexels or hardware pixels is _____ and not subject to change.

131. Therefore, the _____ for these devices is also fixed and does not change.

132. DR dexels (detector elements) are hardware—Their size is fixed and never changes, regardless of detector plate size or _____.

133. DR dexels range from _____ to 200 microns.

134. A 100-micron dexel produces an SF of about ___ LP/mm.

135. Therefore, their inherent sharpness is _____.

136. For example, if a larger DR detector plate is used, technically the matrix size has increased. Yet, the dexels themselves are the _____ size. Therefore, their inherent sharpness is consistent.

137. In an LCD display monitor, each hardware pixel is a _____, composed of the intersection of two flat, transparent wires that conduct electricity (Next Chapter)

138. For a particular manufacturer and model, the size of these pixels is _____.

139. The hardware pixel size sets the _____ resolution with which any image can be displayed on that brand of monitor.

140. For a particular brand, a larger monitor will have more pixels, but the _____ of the pixels is the same. Sharpness is consistent for different size monitors.

141. For a DR detector, collimation of the x-ray beam results in a _____ anatomical area being recorded on the detector plate.

142. This results in a restricted (although magnified) _____-of-view (FOV) displayed on the monitor.

143. Nonetheless, the _____ sharpness of DR is not changed by collimation, because dexel size is unchanged.

144. For a display monitor, _____ of the image results in a smaller anatomical area being displayed.

145. Again, this is a restricted field-of-_____ (FOV) displayed on the monitor.

146. Nonetheless, the inherent sharpness of display monitor itself is not changed, because hardware _____ size is unchanged.

147. To summarize, the hardware elements in DR detectors and display monitors have a fixed size, so these devices have _____ inherent sharpness regardless of changes to matrix size or FOV.

148. A "soft" matrix is a matrix that can be _____ within the physical area of the display.

149. For a soft matrix, pixel size can be _____.

150. For a soft matrix, field-of-view and matrix size _____ change pixel size.

151. For a CR reader, the diameter of the red laser beam can be "collimated" to different widths, changing pixel _____.

152. For a DR detector, dexels are well _____ and their area is fixed.

153. For a CR reader, pixels are round and _____ each other. Pixel size can be changed by effectively "collimating" the area struck by the _____ beam scanning the PSP plate.

154. If the physical area of the displayed image is fixed, the only way to fit a larger matrix with more pixels into the physical area is to make the pixels _____.

Digital Image Acquisition 81

155. This results in _____ sharpness.

156. For a displayed light image, the larger the matrix, the _____ the sharpness.

157. On a display monitor, the "zoom" feature can magnify or _____ the displayed image.

158. Magnification of the displayed image is accomplished only by magnifying each "_____" pixel of the light image.

159. The pixel value for an original single pixel is spread out across a 4-pixel _____ on the monitor.

160. Further magnification spreads it out over a square of _____ hardware pixels.

161. The hardware pixels of the monitor do not change, but the visually apparent pixels of the light image itself are each getting _____.

162. Excessive magnification of the displayed image results in a _____ image as sharpness is lost.

163. On a display monitor, the _____ field-of-view may be selected.

164. For a displayed image, the smaller the smaller the field-of-view, (the more zoom applied), the _____ the sharpness.

165. *Fixed matrix systems* scan by dividing the image into the same number of pixels per _____, regardless of the "effective FOV" created by the IR size or collimation.

166. This causes the sampling frequency to vary based on the size of the image _____. A smaller IR has shorter "rows," pixels must therefore be smaller relative to the image. Smaller IR's present improved sharpness compared to larger imaging plates.

167. *Fixed sampling systems* achieve consistent sharpness by keeping the sampling _____ size the same regardless of the "effective FOV" created by the IR.

168. Most modern CR systems are fixed _____ systems.

169. For light images being displayed on a monitor or being emitted from a PSP plate in a CR reader, pixels are "soft" and the pixel _____ formula applies:

> For a given physical area, Pixel Size = $\dfrac{\text{FOV}}{\text{Matrix}}$

> Practice:
> What is the "soft" pixel size for a 305 mm image (FOV) displayed on a monitor screen with a 1024 X 1024 matrix?

> Solution: $\dfrac{305}{1024}$ = ___ mm pixel size

170. The pixel size formula applies to fixed matrix CR systems. It does NOT apply to fixed _____ CR systems (most modern CR systems).

171. **Summary: Field of View, Matrix Size, and Sharpness:** The _____ spatial resolution of hardware arrays is unaffected by changes in FOV, IR size, collimation, or "zoom," because the physical size of any hardware pixel or dexel is not subject to change.

172. The spatial resolution of a _____ image from a display monitor or PSP plate is affected by FOV and matrix size. The pixel size formula applies in these cases.

173. **Foundational Principle:** Ultimately, it is the size of the _____ or _____ being used to acquire or display the image that determines its sharpness (spatial resolution).

Efficiency of Image Receptors

174. CR phosphor plates and indirect-conversion DR phosphor plates convert energy from x-rays into _____.

175. An average x-ray photon of 30 keV (30,000 volts) can potentially be "split" into 10,000 blue light photons of ___ volts each.

176. STEPS: The phosphor plate must _____ 1) Absorb the x-ray, 2) Convert the energy into light (not heat), and 3) Emit the light toward the AMA. (Most light is emitted in all other directions—Some does not "_____" the plate to reach the IR.

Digital Image Acquisition

177. Materials used for the front panels of image receptor plates, cassettes and x-ray tables must be as _____ as possible while still providing structural protection.

178. The 3 types of efficiency apply to all imaging phosphors are:
    1. _____ Efficiency. (High atomic-number detection layers help).
    2. _____ Efficiency. (A function of the particular _____.
    3. _____ Efficiency

179. In a CR PSP plate, the _____ backing helps direct some light back toward the light guide of the reader.

180. **Indirect-Conversion DR:** Even if only a few percent of the 10,000 light photons emitted per x-ray reach the IR, this would still be _____ light photons.

181. Since blue light photons have only 3 volts of energy, they are not very penetrating and are easily absorbed by the _____ detection layer of the dexel.

182. Because of this increased efficiency, indirect-conversion DR systems require less radiographic _____ than direct-conversion systems, saving patient dose.

183. But direct-conversion systems have higher _____ (because there is no light dispersion). Both systems continue in clinical use, because each has advantages.

184. **Conversion Efficiency of the Active Matrix Array (AMA):** In either type of DR system, once x-ray or light photons are absorbed in a dexel of the AMA, the conversion of this energy into _____ charge is nearly 100%.

185. The "emission" of this signal, the percentage of electrons reaching the capacitors, is also nearly ____%.

186. Thus, conversion and emission efficiency are not substantial concerns for Active Matrix _____.

187. **Detective Quantum Efficiency (DQE)** is measured by physicists as the squared _____ signal-to-noise ratio divided by the squared _____ signal-to-noise ratio:

$$DQE = \frac{SNR^2 \text{ out}}{SNR^2 \text{ in}}$$

188. DQE measures the overall efficiency for converting input exposure data into a useful output _____.

189. No imaging system can achieve a perfect DQE of _____ (100%).

190. At 70 kV, typical DQEs are:
    0.3 (30%) or less for ____ phosphor plates
    0.67 (67%) for _____-conversion DR receptors
    0.77 (77%) for _____-conversion DR receptors

191. High DQE is important, but must be evaluated along with latitude response, sampling methods, display quality and other aspects of the _____.

192. The semiconductor detection surface of a dexel can be primarily sensitive to either: _____ (if made of selenium), OR _____ (if made of silicon).

193. The efficiency factor for any type of dexel (detector element) is measured by physicists as its _____ quantum efficiency (DQE).

194. The percentage of a dexel's square area devoted to the semiconductor detection layer is called the dexel's _____ factor.

195. A higher fill factor provides higher contrast resolution and higher _____-noise ratio (SNR).

196. A current limitation on dexel size is the inability to further miniaturize the _____ and _____.

197. As a result, the smaller the dexel, the _____ the fill factor.

198. With a smaller percentage of detection surface area, an increase in radiographic _____ is necessitated, increasing patient dose.

Digital Sampling and Aliasing

199. For any particular image, certain sampling frequencies can cause geometric artifacts know as Moire patterns or _____.

200. The core cause of all aliasing artifacts is insufficient _____ of high-frequency signals.

201. Aliasing or the Moire artifact is a form of _____.

202. Aliasing appears as false patterns of straight, diagonal, or curved _____.

203. Aliasing patterns emerge in the image whenever there is insufficient sampling of High-_____ digital signals.

204. To prevent aliasing, the Nyquist Theorem states that the sampling frequency must be at least ___ times the spatial frequency of the image being sampled.

205. This is just another way of saying that each _____ of the digital signal must be sampled.

206. (Recall that each cycle consists of 2 pulses, so _____ the frequency simply gives the number of pulses.)

207. If the number of samples taken is less than half the image frequency, _____ lines are created where sampling overlaps the image frequency.

There are several variations on how insufficient sampling can occur:

208. Any time a _____ of a digital image is made (by copy machine, or by camera)

209. Repeated "zooming" magnification of an image on a _____ monitor

210. Insufficient sampling rate in a CR _____.

211. Placing a _____-frequency radiographic grid over a high-frequency digital image

212. Superimposing _____ or other "sampling" devices.

213. In the digital age, this "_____ version" of aliasing is much more common than Moire from grids.

214. Anti-aliasing _____ can reduce the occurrence of electronic aliasing.

215. Use of a _____ grid (such as during a portable procedure) effectively introduces a "sampling" device into the imaging process.

216. The image is "sampled" by the spaces between grid _____.

217. To prevent aliasing, 1) Use a conventional grid with very _____ frequency (expensive), 2) Use special "_____" grid (expensive), OR . . .

218. Use _____ technique. Many anatomical parts can be radiographed non-grid, and *virtual grid software* obviates the need for grids in many cases.

Other Digital Artifacts

219. In DR systems, detector elements can suffer from various electronic faults resulting in dexel _____.

220. Electronic _____ is more common for DR systems than for CR.

221. For CR, the most common source of artifacts is the image _____ plate (scratches, dirt or dust).

222. For CR, ghost images (retained from last exposure) due to incomplete _____.

223. CR artifacts which appear consistently on images from different cassettes are likely the result of problems with the CR _____.

224. Line or column drop-out can result from malfunction of the reader _____ and scanning systems.

225. Dust particles sticking to _____ components in the CR reader can cause pixel drop-out.

226. Dust on optics can delete an entire _____ in the image.

227. Other artifacts can result from:
    _____ failure
    _____ of histogram analysis
    Improper _____ of special features (e.g.,smoothing or EE)
    _____ artifacts.

Chapter 12

DISPLAYING THE DIGITAL IMAGE

1. LCDs have become the predominant type of image _____ monitor in imaging departments.

2. The LCD is attached to a computer that gives the operator the capability of _____ and otherwise manipulating the image as it is viewed.

3. A *workstation* is a fully-equipped computer terminal that can manipulate image quality and permanently _____ changes made into the PAC system.

4. A *diagnostic workstation* is used for diagnosis. A radiologist's *class 1* workstation requires two _____-resolution (2000 x 2000 pixel) display monitors for comparison views.

5. In addition, a typical PC display monitor and computer are used to _____ the images displayed on the high-resolution monitors and associated patient files.

6. A typical radiographer's workstation has a single, lower-resolution *class* __ display monitor –1000 x 1000 pixels.

7. A *display station* is limited to image display, with no ability to _____ change the image saved into the PACS system.

8. A display station is ____ resolution.

9. Display stations can be strategically placed throughout a hospital and in affiliated clinics to allow doctors ready _____ to images.

The Liquid Crystal Display (LCD) Monitor

10. *Liquid crystal display (LCD)* monitors work on the basis of the _____ of light.

11. Polarizing "lenses" use long, slender, aligned _____ of iodine molecules which act as a _____.

12. Only those light waves whose electrical component vibrates _____ to these chains of molecules can penetrate through.

13. Perpendicular ones are _____.

14. By placing _____ polarizing lenses perpendicular to each other, _____ light will be blocked. This arrangement is used for LCD monitor screens.

15. In panels' normal position, their string molecules of the two panels are _____ to each other.

16. The LCD process involves "tricking" these layers into allowing light to pass through when we wish, by using a special material in between them which _____ the light.

17. This material consists of _____ liquid crystals (usually of hydrogenated amorphous silicon).

18. The term *nematic* means they have a long, thread-like shape, and tend to _____ parallel with each other.

19. The term *liquid* means they are able to _____ around each other, even though they have crystalline structure.

20. Each polarizing plate includes a layer of thin, flat wires to conduct electricity that are also _____.

21. Running perpendicular to each other, each junction of wires forms a hardware _____ in the monitor screen.

22. When you touch the LCD screen, you are directly touching these transparent pixel _____.

23. Excessive pressure can _____ them. Most "dead" pixels occur from this type of abuse.

24. At each pixel, front and back electrodes have fine _____ etched into their polymer surfaces.

25. The "threads" of liquid crystals tend to _____ with these scratches in the surfaces of the electrodes when the electrodes are *not* charged.

26. Scratches on the front and back electrodes are _____ to each other.

27. This causes the liquid crystals to line up in spiral pattern _____ 90 degrees between the two plates.

28. Light _____ the orientation of the crystals.

29. This allows light to pass through _____ filters.

30. The pixel is considered to be in the "on state" allowing light to pass through, as long as no electrical _____ is applied to the pixel electrodes.

31. When an electrical charge is applied to the pixel, the nematic crystals align to the _____, all parallel to each other.

32. The twisting effect is lost, light is _____ and unable to pass through the 2nd polarizing filter.

33. Without the twisting effect, the result is a _____ spot in the image.

34. When electrical charge is applied to the pixel, it is considered to be shut "_____" (!)

35. Different voltages applied cause more or less twisting, resulting in various _____ shades.

36. To the side of the polarizing panels, electronics control the electrical current to each _____ of pixels of the active matrix _____ (AMA) of an LCD panel.

Displaying the Digital Image

37. The one remaining need is to supply a source of light to pass through the panels: For a _____-matrix LCD, such as a typical wrist watch or calculator, normal room lighting or sunlight is _____ off a shiny surface behind the filter plates.

38. A source of sidelighting can also be provided for when it is dark—this also reflects off of the _____ surface.

39. The displays needed for computer monitors and imaging applications must be much _____ and provide higher contrast and resolution than provided by passive-matrix LCDs.

40. To achieve adequate brightness, these display monitors use LEDs (light-emitting diodes) or _____ bulbs as a backlighting source.

41. A pair of very thin fluorescent _____ can be mounted to the side of the monitor.

42. Several special _____ disperse light from the side-mounted fluorescent bulbs evenly across the screen.

43. Compared to slow-responding passive LCDs used in watches and calculators, much _____ *response* and *refresh* times are necessary for display monitors.

44. To achieve these, the _____-matrix LCD (AMLCD) was developed, in which each pixel has its own dedicated thin-film transistor (TFT).

45. This allows entire _____ of pixels to be read out one at a time, rather than single pixels one at a time.

46. *Response time* is the time for a pixel to _____ brightness.

47. *Refresh time* is the time to construct the next image _____.

48. Various digital processing operations can be applied by the _____.

49. But, too much digital processing can cause *input lag*, _____ display.

50. Truly dead pixels appear as permanent _____ spots.

51. Permanent dark spots on the monitor screen are "_____" pixels that are constantly receiving electrical charge.

52. A monitor should be replaced if there are more than ___ bad pixels overall, more than 3 in any 1cm circle, or more than 3 adjacent to each other.

LCD Image Quality

Advantages of the LCD include:

53. No distortion or variation in _____

54. No glare and minimal _____

55. Uniform _____ with no flicker

Disadvantages of the LCD include:

56. _____ (upon close inspection, dark lines between pixels can be seen)

57. Limited contrast from an inability to produce "true _____" (as older CRTs could).

58. There is always some light _____ from backlighting elements, reducing contrast.

59. Brightness is both _____-dependent and temperature-dependent.

60. A 15-minute _____-___ time is required when first energized.

61. Limited _____ angle due to brightness loss.

62. Luminous intensity drops off as viewing _____ of the observer is increased.

63. Observers must try to stand as "head-on" as possible, directly in _____ of the monitor.

64. Maximum sharpness, i.e., inherent resolution capability, is ultimately determined by the size of the LCD's _____ pixels.

65. Or the size of the _____ used to record the latent image, if they are larger than the LCD pixels.

66. (The _____ of "soft" pixels in the actual displayed light image is relative and can be changed by magnification or zooming. In this chapter, however, we are concerned only with the hardware pixels of the LCD monitor itself)

67. For a particular manufacturer, these are of _____ size.

68. The smaller they are, the _____ the inherent sharpness of the monitor.

69. Dot _____ or pixel _____ is the distance between the centers of any two adjacent hardware pixels.

70. The smaller the dot pitch, the smaller the pixels, and the higher the inherent _____ of the device.

71. Assuming a fixed physical size of display area, the more pixels in the matrix, the _____ they must be, and the sharper the resolution.

72. Generally, the pixel size on a computer monitor is about 0.2 mm, and for a high-resolution Class 1 monitor it can be as small as ____ mm.

73. Focal spot sizes are 0.5–0.6 mm for the small FS and 1.0–1.2 mm for the large FS. Due to the typical SOD and OID used, penumbra width is roughly 1/10th the focal spot size, or 0.12 mm for the large FS. This rivals the _____ size for the LCD.

74. Therefore, it is possible on some procedures that using the large focal spot improperly could result in more _____ than the display monitor produces.

75. *Luminance* is the _____ of light emitted from a source such as an LCD.

76. List the three most common units for luminance:
    _____
    _____
    _____

77. To measure brightness, we must define the size of the _____ from which we will gather light.

78. Light from an LCD fills a _____-shaped hemisphere.

79. We divide the volume of space within this hemisphere into _____.

80. One steradian is a _____ with a radius "r" from the source of light, whose base has an area = r^2

81. Using this formula, there are ~12.5 steradians in a sphere. There are just over ___ steradians in a hemisphere.

82. The *candela* measures the total rate of light emitted by a typical candle in ____ directions.

83. The *lumen* refers to the brightness of that light within _____ steradian.

84. A light source with one candela of brightness generates one _____ per steradian around it.

85. One lumen per steradian is about 0.0015 _____ of power per steradian. (Since the watt expresses the energy rate per second, time is already taken into account in the formula.)

86. The photometer is a device used to measure the light _____ from a display monitor.

87. It uses the _____ effect to generate electrical current and display the read-out.

88. Read-out may be in lumens, lux, or candela per square _____.

89. The American College of Radiology (ACR) requires a minimum brightness capability for radiologic display systems of _____ lumens (Lm). The typical range preferred by radiologists is 500–600 Lm, and the maximum capability for most LCDs is _____ Lm.

90. In a diagnostic reading room, ambient lighting must be _____ to a point where both diffuse reflectance and specular reflectance are below any noticeable level.

91. LCDs generally have low _____. Task Group 18 of the AAPM has published guidelines for maximum illuminance in reading rooms.

Displaying the Digital Image 95

92. Diffuse reflectance is the cumulative effect of ambient _____ lighting across the surface area of the display monitor screen.

93. Specular reflectance refers to the reflection of a specific, localized light _____ such as a light bulb.

94. *Illuminance* refers to the rate of light striking a _____, or how well objects in our field of view are illuminated by a light source.

95. For example, the *luminance* of a desk lamp _____ a paper on the desk in front of it.

96. The effect of ambient room lighting on the surface of an LCD monitor screen, including the reflectance off the screen, is the result of _____ in the room.

97. Excessive illuminance reduces the apparent visual _____ of the displayed image.

98. The unit for illuminance is the ____, defined as 1 lumen per square meter of surface area
$$1 \text{ lux} = 1 \text{ Lm} / m^2$$

99. Typical illuminance levels:
    Direct sunlight: 105 lux
    Full moonlight: 10 lux
    Typical office lighting: 75-_____ lux
    Radiologic reading room lighting: 2-25 lux

100. Ambient lighting for a radiologic reading room must never exceed ____ normal office lighting, or 25 lux.

101. Viewing _____ dependence can be measured using a photometer at increasing angles off perpendicular to the LCD, to compare monitors.

The Nature of Display Pixels

102. For an LCD, each hardware pixel has a roughly square shape and definite area about the size of a 10-point font _____.

103. In a color monitor, each pixel must be capable of displaying the entire _____ of colors in the spectrum.

104. To achieve this, three _____ are used, yellow-green, red, and blue. All three must be lit together to produce white.

105. In constructing an image for display, we define a pixel as the _____ screen element that can display ALL of the gray levels (or colors) within the dynamic range of the system.

106. A pixel consists of a group of _____ subpixels.

107. _____ (black-and-white) display monitors are sufficient for most medical imaging purposes.

108. Each pixel actually consists of 18 individual bar-like segments, three segments makes a domain, a pair of domains makes a _____.

109. For a monochrome display, each subpixel can be treated as a separately _____ element by the computer, producing entire range of gray levels from black to white, acting as a _____ pixel.

110. The darkness of each subpixel can be controlled by varying the _____ applied to It.

111. Thus, for a monochrome display monitor, we acquire 3 functional pixels in the same _____ that a single pixel in a color monitor requires.

112. This leads to ___ times higher resolution than a similar color monitor.

113. The display monitor is typically much more _____ in both resolution and dynamic range (bit depth) than the digital image processing system of the computer.

114. This is why class 1 monitors for radiologist's diagnosis station are so _____.

115. It is also why radiographers must be careful about judging images displayed on a class ___ workstation monitor.

116. A poor quality monitor can effectively _____ the sharpness already achieved during image acquisition and processing.

Chapter 13

ARCHIVING PATIENT IMAGES AND INFORMATION

Picture Archiving and Communication Systems (PACS)

1. Every imaging system must include:
   First, a machine for image _____
   Second, equipment for image _____
   Third, devices for image display and _____

2. The image must be converted from an analog image to a digital image (using an ADC) between acquisition and processing, and back from a _____ to an _____ image (using a DAC) just prior to display.

3. *PACS* stands for *Picture _____ and Communication System.*

4. Through digitization, images from ____ different modalities within a department can be stored on magnetic tapes, magnetic discs or optical discs

5. The PACS server provides a long-term image storage system that can . . .
   a. _____ images
   b. _____ images for viewing
   c. _____ images to remote locations

6. Service Class Users (SCUs) include image acquisition and display stations in clinics and hospitals that need to _____ the system.

7. Service Class Providers (SCPs) include all _____ devices that manage storage and distribution of images, and PACS workstations.

8. A PACS is actually a local area _____ or *LAN*.

9. The central control computer _____ the flow of images and data between:

   a. Acquisition stations from various _____ modalities
   b. The _____ Information System (RIS)
   c. The _____ Information System (HIS)
   d. _____ in clinics, hospital departments, and radiologist homes.

10. The PACS _____ can store over 1 million images en masse.

11. The PACS stores all these images using magnetic or optical _____, stacks of over 100 discs.

12. Some systems employ wide area networks (WANs) to allow access at _____ locations.

13. Fiber optic technology _____ data at very high speeds.

14. The PACS control computer must be compatible to interface with all different _____ of medical equipment in the HIS, the RIS, acquisition stations and workstations.

15. A _____ high-level computer language was needed.

16. In the 1980s, a joint committee of the ACR and the NEMA developed the _____ standard.

17. *DICOM* stands for *Digital Imaging and _____ in Medicine*.

18. DICOM specifies only the _____ behavior of the various devices, not the specific architecture or terminology between different makes of devices.

19. The main function of the PAC system is to act as a _____.

20. Sample DICOM Commands include:

   a. DICOM *get* _____ can generate lists of patients or studies from the HIS or RIS.
   b. DICOM _____/*retrieve* can search out specific images or studies.
   c. DICOM *send* transmits data to the _____
   d. DICOM *print*

Archiving Patient Images and Information 99

21. _____ is extensive, detailed information stored "behind the image" for every image.

22. Metadata includes:

   a. _____ on the patient
   b. _____ used for the procedure
   c. Image parameters and _____ used

23. Key items of interest to caregivers are made easily accessible at the touch of a button while the image is displayed, as a DICOM _____.

24. A true header is displayed as a bar along the top of the image, a summary of _____ data.

25. Items in the metadata each have a universal DICOM _____ identifier at the left, followed by a description of the type of information being given, then the actual setting, status or value being used.

26. The PACS system allows _____ of the image:

   a. _____ brightness and contrast
   b. _____ & minification
   c. _____

27. Web-based PACS allow _____ access

28. Encryption software helps protect _____.

29. *Image* _____ is necessary for cost-effective long-term storage because image file sizes can be up to 4–5 Megabytes each for CR and DR radiographs, 15 MB each for MRI images, and 25 MB each for CT images.

30. At 200 radiographs, 100 MRI images, and 100 CT images per day, this comes to _____ Gigabytes per month.

31. Lossy compression ratios, above 10:1, result in irreversible loss of spatial resolution (sharpness), _____ for medical diagnosis.

32. _____ compression ratios, defined as less than 8:1, have been deemed "visually acceptable" by radiologists.

33. Image storage capacity must be _____ for workstations.

34. To make room for newly acquired studies, the station must _____ images on regular time-frame.

35. For CR, DR, CT, MRI, NM and US units, usually erasure is done __ hours after acquisition.

36. For quality assurance stations and for radiologists' level 1 workstations, usually erasure is done after ___ days.

37. Within the PACS server, _____ or *on-line* storage is temporary and uses optical discs or magnetic media for any file recently accessed.

38. Archive (long-term) storage uses jukeboxes, often in a _____ location.

39. It can take more than 5 _____ to access a file from archive storage.

40. *Prefetching:* During the night, the system automatically searches the HIS and RIS for _____ images and records for patients scheduled the following day, and brings them to workstations for immediate access.

41. Different _____ are followed according to the type of procedure.

42. For example, for a chest procedure, the *prefetching* program may bring up the most _____ PA and lateral chest views.

43. Radiologists' workstations include intelligent, _____ "hanging" protocols, decision support tools (e.g., CAD), and special reprocessing features.

44. Three approaches for clinics to access the PACS:
    a. Install PACS _____ at the site
    b. Install PACS _____

45. Integrate PACS images into patient's electronic records in the HIS. This limits _____ of the image to display adjustments only.

46. The highest viewing _____ and most powerful options for image manipulation require PACS workstations.

47. *DICOM* _____ should be included on CD or DVD along with any images sent to clinical sites.

Archiving Patient Images and Information 101

48. Using the viewer software to display the images _____ image quality and manipulation features.

49. Without a DICOM viewer, monitors and software at the clinical site can severely compromise image _____.

50. Typical compression for attachments _____ image resolution.

51. A special URL (uniform _____ locator) can be generated that allows clinicians _____-access to images stored with full file size, along with the DICOM viewer software, on a server.

52. *RAID* stands for "_____ Array of Independent Disks."

53. A RAID system distributes copies of the same data files across several computer hard drives which are _____ of each other.

54. This assures that medical information or images are not _____ by electrical failure, file corruption or software failure in a single system.

55. Before PACS, loss of medical documents was estimated at between 5 and ___ percent.

56. Storage Area _____ (SANs) protect against loss of files from _____ disasters.

57. A SAN is a sub-network connecting several storage devices at remote geographic _____ or other clinical sites.

58. Note that SAN components are connected in _____, so that if one component fails, connections between other components are not broken.

59. An _____ number, assigned by the RIS for each exam, and should be displayed in the DICOM header for every view.

60. The HIS also assigns a *unique* number to each _____.

61. The PAC system verifies _____ between these numbers prior to storage and upon access.

Medical Imaging Informatics

62. *Medical informatics* is the effective use of medical data, information and knowledge to improve healthcare through _____ computer servers and workstations.

63. In medical imaging, informatics improves management and _____ of images.

64. This includes _____, accuracy, and real-time interactive functionality of imaging services.

65. *Health Level Seven Standard (HL7)* is an ongoing publication by Health Level Seven International since 1987 to _____ the way that health information is retrieved, exchanged, integrated, and shared.

66. HL7 is to medical information what _____ is to medical images.

67. The *Electronic Medical Record (EMR)* is the digital version of a patient's _____ for a clinical practice.

68. The *EMR* includes lab and pathology results, radiology _____, and nurse and physician notes.

69. The EMR provides efficient _____ of information, and more effective patient care.

70. For example, the EMR can add _____ reminders for screening procedures and check-ups.

71. PACS have begun to _____ with EMRs to make images more accessible to referring physicians.

72. The *Electronic Health Record (EHR)* is a goal of modern healthcare, a complete _____ medical history designed to be shared between healthcare providers.

73. Whereas, the *EMR* is maintained within a _____ clinical practice.

74. In the USA, _____ (the *Healthcare Insurance Portability and Accountability Act*) regulates patient privacy rights.

75. Many healthcare providers and insurance companies now make entire EMR's accessible to the patient via the _____.

76. Healthcare providers are held accountable by law (HIPAA) to maintain each patient's _____ through record-keeping, written communications, internet and electronic media, and _____ communications.

77. Radiographers must take special _____ in all these settings.

78. List the *three* elements of security for medical records:

    a. _____
    b. _____
    c. _____

79. *Privacy:* Ensures access to medical information _____ to those for whom it was intended.

80. *Authentication:* Allows senders and recipients of medical information to _____ each others' identities.

81. *Integrity:* Guarantees incoming information has not been _____.

82. A *firewall* is a router, computer, or network that provides system _____.

83. The *HIS (Hospital Information System)* is an "_____" computer system integrating all information flow within hospital or clinic.

84. The HIS is comprised of _____ Information Systems *(CISs),* such as the RIS, and _____ Information Systems *(AISs).*

85. *Protocols* are _____ that facilitate exchange of data between the nodes of a computer network.

86. A *TCP* (_____ *Control Protocol*) divides information to be sent into "packets."

87. *IP* (_____ *Protocol*) governs the actual transmission.

88. *Routers* use these protocols to connect _____ and the internet.

89. A *LAN (local area network)* used within a single organization is an _____.

90. _____ is the protocol used within a PACS.

Chapter 14

DIGITAL FLUOROSCOPY

1. *Fluoroscopy* is the production of dynamic (moving) radiographic images in _____ or as they occur.

2. Fluoroscopy was invented by Thomas Edison in 1896, just ____ year after Roentgen discovered x-rays.

3. The original fluoroscope consisted of a metal cone with a _____ screen in the bottom and a small viewing window in the top.

4. For "open fluoroscopy," a large intensifying screen was positioned behind the patient in a completely darkened room—the radiologist had to _____-adapt his eyes to the very dim image.

5. Exposure to both the patient and to the radiologist (whose head was directly in the remnant x-ray beam) was _____.

6. The *electronic image intensifier tube,* invented by John Coltman in the late 1940s, converted the x-ray image into an _____ beam that could be accelerated and focused for intensification.

7. This dramatically reduced the mA required, saving patient _____.

8. Today there are two types of fluoroscopes: The *Dynamic Flat Panel Detector (DFPD)* uses the same flat panel detector (FPD) technology as direct-conversion ____ (Chapter 11), but with _____ dexels and electronics to accommodate moving images.

9. The acquired electronic image is sent directly to _____.

10. The *Image Intensifier* is older technology. Since it emits a light image, a recording _____ must be mounted on top.

Image Recording from an Image Intensifier Tube

11. The Image Intensifier converts the incoming image into an electron beam that is _____ and _____.

12. The output phosphor of the tube then converts the electron energy into a _____ image emitted from the top.

13. The light image is transmitted through a bundle of _____ fibers directly to a 2.5 cm CCD or CMOS camera.

14. *CCD* stands for *charge-_____ device*.

15. CMOS stands for *Complimentary Metal-Oxide _____*.

16. The CCD is a small, flat plate only 1/2-inch in size for the home cam-corder, or 1 inch for fluoroscopy. Its sensitive surface is made of crystalline _____, a semiconductor.

17. When light photons ionize molecules in the silicon layer, freed electrons drift upward toward the dielectric layer, and positively-charged holes drift downward to a _____ of microscopic electrodes.

18. Hole drift actually consists of a series of electrons moving up to fill each vacancy in the molecule layer above, in sequence, such that the _____ itself, the "hole," appears to drift in the opposite direction.

19. This is very similar to direct-conversion ____ dexels (Chapter 11).

20. When a "hole" reaches an electrode, it pulls an electron from it, creating a _____ charge on the electrode which can be measured by the circuit.

21. Each electrode is connected to a storage capacitor and a thin-film _____ (TFT) that acts as an electronic gate (or switch).

22. Rows and columns of these TFTs form an active matrix _____ (AMA) which holds the "latent" image until it is electronically read out.

Digital Fluoroscopy

23. The electronic signal, as it drains from each row of the CCD, is boosted by an electronic _____.

24. CCDs achieve very high _____.

25. A typical 2.5 cm CCD has a matrix of 2048 X 2048 pixels, making each pixel only 14 microns in _____.

26. This amazing level of miniaturization is possible because: For the CCD, each TFT constitutes a _____.

27. Whereas for DR, each dexel constitutes a pixel. The TFT is just a _____ of the dexel.

28. Rather than individual dexels each having its own detection surface as a DR detector does, for the CCD, the entire active matrix array of TFTs underlies a _____ detection surface.

Charge-Coupled Devices (CCDs) have:

29. High spatial resolution (sharpness)
High detective quantum efficiency (DQE), allowing _____ technique and patient dose

30. High signal-to-noise ratio (SNR)
Long _____ range (3000:1, ideal for fluoro)

31. Twice the frame _____ of conventional TV cameras: 60 frames per second

32. The *CMOS* consists of two MOSFET transistors (one positive, one negative) stacked together to form an electronic logic _____.

33. Initially used in integrated circuits for computers, it was found a CMOS could _____ electric charge from a layer of silicon above just like CCDs.

34. Initially very poor for imaging, recent advances have led to a _____ of CMOS for imaging.

35. For CMOS, the initial light image _____ is identical to that of the CCD:

36. Both use the _____ effect.

37. Both collect these electrons as an electrical charge in a layer of _____ below.

38. The main difference is that the CCD consists of a single, _____ detection surface, with an underlying active matrix array made up only of TFTs.

39. Whereas the CMOS sensor consists of individual dexels, _____ of which has its own separate detection surface.

40. In the CCD, since the AMA is overlaid by a continuous sensitive surface, nearly _____ of the surface is dedicated to light capture.

41. For the CMOS, all the electronics in each dexel take _____ away from the sensitive surface area.

42. The CMOS has a lower _____ factor, which increases noise.

43. CMOS: has more _____ in each dexel even than a DR detector. (A TFT, an amplifier, a noise correction circuit, and a digitization circuit.

44. CMOS has a lower fill factor than even ____.

45. In the CCD, each TFT in the underlying AMA (left) effectively becomes a _____. These are much _____ than the dexels of the CMOS (right), resulting in higher sharpness for the CCD.

46. Improvements have now made CMOS competitive with CCDs: CMOS consumes 1/100th the power, is very inexpensive, and has higher speed due to high conversion _____ of its electronics.

47. CCDs have higher _____ resolution.

48. CMOS has higher _____ resolution.

49. The _____ of data is also different between the CCD and the CMOS:

50. In the CCD, an _____ stream of charge flows to a corner of the AMA where it is digitized and separated into individual pixels.

51. In the CMOS, each charge is already separated (digitized) at the original _____.

Digital Fluoroscopy

Dynamic Flat-Panel Detectors (DFPDs)

52. *Dynamic Flat-Panel Detectors (DFPDs)* are replacing image intensifier _____.

53. DFPDs use the same types of detector elements as direct-conversion and indirect-conversion ____ (Chapter 11), only with larger dexel sizes.

54. As with DR, there are two types of DFPDs: _____-capture detectors that use an active matrix array (AMA) of amorphous selenium dexels, and _____-capture detectors that use an AMA of amorphous silicon dexels.

55. For *indirect-capture,* the dexels are positioned under a _____ layer of phosphorescent material.

56. The phosphor can be cesium iodide, OR _____.

57. Cesium iodide can be formed into _____-shaped crystals that direct most emitted light straight downward to improve sharpness.

58. Gadolinium crystals are turbid, meaning they are a _____ that cannot be shaped into rods.

59. Gadolinium detectors have slightly less resolution but are _____.

Optional Review: Direct DFP Detectors:

60. Upon ionization by x-rays, electrons freed from molecules drift upward, while positively-charged _____ in the molecules drift downward to the negative electrode.

61. Positive charge, accumulated on the storage capacitors of each TFT, constitute a "_____ image" in the active matrix array (AMA).

Optional Review: Indirect DFP Detectors:

62. A phosphor layer is placed over the AMA, x-rays cause the phosphor to _____.

63. Light photons striking the AMA below have the _____ effect on amorphous silicon as x-rays do on amorphous selenium.

64. Observation of moving fluoroscopic images does not require the _____ level of spatial resolution that static (still) images do.

65. Static flat panel detectors (FPDs) used for DR have a dexel size of 100–150 microns, (0.1–0.15 mm). Dynamic flat panel detectors (DFPDs) used for digital fluoroscopy have larger pixel sizes of _____-_____ microns.

66. Dual use digital systems have 100–150 micron dexels for high-resolution "spot" images, then for fluoroscopy mode they _____ together groups of 4 dexels each to form an effective pixel with dimensions of 200–300 microns.

67. This allows reduced _____ and patient dose during fluoroscopy.

68. Typical dimensions of entire DFPD panel = 43 x 43 cm (17 x 17 inches) with matrix sizes up to _____ dexels.

69. Indirect-conversion systems produce a resolution of about _____ LP/mm.

70. The _____ layer (the AMA), not the scintillation phosphor, is the limiting factor for sharpness.

71. Although the Image Intensifier initially produces twice the sharpness (5 LP/mm), a CCD or CMOS camera mounted atop it brings this resolution back _____ to a level comparable to the DFPD.

72. Depending on manufacturer quality, _____ system may be sharper overall.

73. With an image intensifier, changing to a smaller the field-of-view results in higher sharpness. With a DFPD, sharpness is _____ regardless of the FOV used.

74. After each frame, a light-emitting diode (LED) array below the detector produces a bright microsecond flash to "_____" residual electrical charge that would result in "ghost images."

75. Grids for DFPDs have their lead lines running _____ to prevent aliasing artifacts (Chap. 4).

76. Lower _____ (6:1) grids can be used for digital fluoroscopy, allowing reduced technique and lower patient dose.

Digital Fluoroscopy

77. *Advantages* of DFPDs over Image Intensifiers include freedom from various forms of distortion, they are smaller, lighter, and easier to use, they require less power, have a higher signal-to-noise ratio, and extended _____ range.

78. *Disadvantages* of DFPDs include expense, possibility of _____ pixels, and they may have lower sharpness.

Reducing Patient Dose

79. *Intermittent fluoroscopy* is using a series of _____ visual checks, rather than continuous fluoroscopy.

80. This dramatically reduces _____ exposure to the patient.

81. *Intermittent fluoroscopy* is the most important way to limit patient exposure during _____ studies.

82. A 5-minute timer is designed to remind the operator when _____ beam-on time is becoming excessive.

83. DO NOT _____ THE TIMER BEFORE IT SOUNDS.

84. In recent years there have arisen several cases of severe radiation _____ and lesions to patients from cardiovascular and surgical C-arm procedures.

85. "Last Image _____ devices, keeping the last image displayed on the monitor until the next exposure is made, help avoid _____ fluoroscoping and have been shown to reduce cumulative patient exposure as much as 50%–80%.

86. A second monitor allows subtracted images or images other than the most recent to be kept on _____.

87. In pulsed fluoroscopy mode, short _____ of radiation are used to produce individual frames.

88. Substantial radiation dose is saved while the beam is shut off between _____.

89. To the human eye, no _____ is apparent at frame rates above 18 frames per second.

90. Therefore, any radiation used to produce more than 18 frames per second is _____.

91. On flat panel C-arm units, mA must be _____ from 2 to 20 mA for sufficient exposure per frame.

92. Still, a _____ reduction in patient dose can be achieved because of extremely short frame exposure times.

93. _____-frequency generators are required to achieve fast interrogation and extinction times.

94. *Interrogation Time* is the time required for x-ray tube to be _____ on.

95. *Extinction Time* is the time required for x-ray tube to be switched _____.

96. Digital units can _____ interpolated frames between actual exposed frames to produce a continuous-looking image.

97. This allows us to reduce the actual exposure frame rate to 15 frames per second, cutting patient exposure in _____.

98. Even 7.5 fps can be used for procedures not requiring _____ resolution.

99. _____ of the x-ray beam spares the patient radiation exposure between frames.

100. Lower frame rates than realtime, (15 or 7.5 fps rather than 30 fps) can be used in conjunction with digital memory to provide a _____-looking image.

101. On some units, further reduction in patient dose can be achieved by reducing the pulse _____ for each frame.

102. Pulse Width is the individual _____ time for each frame exposure.

103. Selecting 3 milliseconds rather than the typical 6 ms, patient dose can again be cut to _____.

104. Newer units combine high mA pulsed mode with special copper _____ to achieve high image quality with low dose.

Chapter 15

QUALITY CONTROL FOR DIGITAL EQUIPMENT

1. *Quality Assurance* is a _____ philosophy that encompasses all aspects of patient care, image production, and image interpretation.

2. *Quality Control* usually refers to calibration and monitoring of _____, and is part of a quality assurance program.

3. Several tests can be performed by the staff radiographer. Some tests are more advanced or require special equipment, and should be done by a medical _____.

4. Radiographers can monitor sudden changes in field uniformity, erasure thoroughness, intrinsic noise and spatial resolution by _____ checks.

Monitoring of Digital X-Ray Units

5. Field Uniformity: Digital detectors are all _____ non-uniform.

6. Digital _____ makes corrections.

7. For an artifact noted repeatedly in same spot, for DR, the _____ plate is suspect. For CR, the _____ and phosphor plate are suspect.

8. For a CR artifact appearing with different cassettes, the CR _____ is suspect.

9. For a *field uniformity* test, take a _____-field exposure with no object in the beam at a moderate technique.

Quality Control for Digital Equipment

10. Thoroughly _____ the CR cassette prior to test exposure. (DR systems automatically erase the detector between exposures.)

11. Open collimation to cover the entire field, and use a long 180 cm SID to minimize anode _____ effect.

12. Visually scan the resulting image for dexel or pixel _____.

13. On the monitor, do not adjust the contrast above normal settings—_____ image will appear non-uniform at high contrast.

14. To measure field density (brightness), use a photometer in 4 _____ and center for comparison.

15. *Intrinsic (Dark) Noise* is _____ noise in the DR detector not related to dexel drop-out, or in the CR phosphor plate not related to the reader.

16. To test for dark noise, erase and then _____ process a single plate without exposing it to an x-ray beam.

17. Scan the resulting image for any unusual amounts of mottle or noise compared to a _____ image.

18. *Ghost images* can indicate:
    1. _____ in the reader are burned out
    2. Loss of lamp intensity in the reader
    3. Too short _____ to lamps in the reader

19. Ghost images can also occur from extreme overexposure during the _____ procedure (when residual electric charge is trapped).

20. To test for ghost images, expose the imaging plate with a step-wedge or other object made of homogeneous material in the beam, (and process if CR). Immediately re-expose the same plate _____ the object in the beam and with 1 inch (2.5 cm) collimation in from each edge. Scan the resulting image for any ghost image of the object.

21. For DR systems, ghosting is also known as "_____ effect."

22. For DR, it is caused by trapped residual electrical _____ that is released only slowly over time.

23. Indirect-conversion systems have more image _____ than direct-conversion systems.

24. To check for changes in sharpness, a flat wire _____ can be exposed, and the image examined for any distortion or blur.

25. Take a _____ image, then test every 6 months.

26. A line-pair template can be used to measure _____ (Chapter 3).

Monitoring of Electronic Image Display Systems

27. The display monitor is the _____ link in the imaging chain. Poor display quality can lead to misdiagnosis!

28. Consistency _____ all monitors within a workstation is essential. All should have the same luminance, be set at the same contrast, and be cleaned monthly.

29. Standards for electronic medical images are available from _____ Part 14. Guidelines and tests are available from several groups, including the AAPM (American Association of Physicists in Medicine), SMPTE (Society of Motion Picture and Television Engineers), and the ACR (American College of Radiology).

30. Class 1 display monitors used for _____ are subject to much more stringent guidelines than Class 2 monitors.

31. Class ___ display monitors may be used for display and a limited amount of image manipulation, but not for documented diagnosis.

32. *Luminance* and *contrast* tests should be performed _____.

33. *Maximum luminance* can be checked with a _____ over the brightest area of any test pattern. Compare with baseline over time.

34. The ACR requires minimum of _____ lumens (Lm) for image display. Radiologists prefer 600 Lm, most LCDs can achieve 800.

35. Recommended luminance is _____ Lm minimum for any LCD.

36. *Luminance response* is a monitor's ability to accurately display _____ shades or levels of brightness from a test pattern.

37. *Luminance response* is essentially identical to a _____ test.

38. On the SMPTE test pattern for luminance response (contrast), adjacent squares in the outer ring should all be _____ (from each other).

39. For the *double squares* marked 0/5% and 95/100%, the _____ squares should be distinguishable. The 50% squares should match.

40. Adjacent squares should measure 10% difference between each other on a photometer, within ___% accuracy.

41. DICOM standards define a Grayscale Standard Display Function (GSDF) based on human perception, with increments of brightness called JND's (Just _____ differences).

42. The AAPM recommends that luminance response should fall within ___% of the GSDF standard.

43. *Luminance* _____ is defined as the maximum luminance divided by minimum luminance.

44. An LCD is not capable of producing a _____ black level while it is energized. This can be seen in a completely darkened room.

45. LCDs have a relatively _____ luminance ratio.

46. Typical LCD luminance ratio falls between 300 and 600. Make baseline, measurement, compare for deterioration over _____.

47. On the SMPTE universal test pattern, black-on-white and white-on-black _____ are used to measure LR.

48. *Luminance uniformity* is the consistency of am single brightness level displayed _____ different areas of the screen.

49. The AAPM recommends that luminance uniformity not deviate more than 30% from the _____.

50. Luminance Uniformity is checked at ___ locations across the screen.

51. The two types of *reflectance* are _____ *reflectance* from ambient room lighting, and _____ reflectance from specific, localized light sources (see Chapter 12).

52. In a diagnostic reading room, ambient _____ must be dimmed to a point where both diffuse reflectance and specular reflectance are below any noticeable level.

53. Reading room lighting should never be more than 25 lux, never more than ___ typical office lighting, which is about 100 lux.

54. The main impact of noise is in reducing image _____.

55. No _____ guidelines have been published for acceptable levels of noise in the electronic radiographic image, nor are the expected because . . .

56. (As explained in Chapter 9), a certain amount of mottle can be _____ to the radiologist in the interest of reducing patient dose.

57. Noise should generally be kept as low as possible, but some noise is inevitable and becomes a secondary consideration in comparison with more important objectives in patient care such as reducing patient _____.

58. Both the ACR and the AAPM recommend a minimum resolution for electronically displayed images of _____ LP/mm.

59. On any test pattern for spatial resolution, series of high-contrast bars of diminishing width are used: Horizontal bars measure _____ resolution. Vertical bars measure _____ resolution.

60. The universal SMPTE pattern has resolution bars in 5 locations: _____ and 4 corners.

61. Each series consists of a set of high-contrast bars and a set of _____-contrast bars.

62. The _____ set of clear bars defines the resolution in LP/mm from a table.

Quality Control for Digital Equipment

63. For most LCDs, one pixel is just the size of a 12-point font _____ or the dot of an "i."

64. A magnifying glass may be used to initially find it, but it should then be visible to the "_____ eye."

65. A defect smaller than this would be caused by the failure of a _____.

66. A _____ glass is necessary to see a faulty subpixel.

67. Failure of any one of the 6 _____ making up a subpixel constitutes a bad subpixel, apparent on close inspection as a smaller defect.

68. A truly _____ pixel appears as a white spot against a solid black background.

69. A _____ "flat field" image must be created for this test.

70. A stuck pixel appears as a _____ spot against a solid white background.

71. A stuck pixel is being continuously supplied with _____.

72. Although a dead or stuck pixel can sometimes be fixed by gently massaging it with the fleshy fingertip, pixels can also be damaged by _____ pressure (as from a fingernail), so this is not recommended for expensive class 1 monitors.

73. The AAPM recommends failing QC for a monitor that has more than 15 bad pixels across the entire screen, more than 3 bad pixels within any 1-cm circle, or more than 3 bad _____ pixels anywhere on the screen.

74. It is not unusual for any LCD to have _____ bad pixels.

75. Class 1 monitors used by radiologists for diagnosis should be "_____ perfect." Class 2 standards are lower.

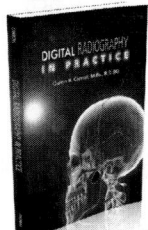

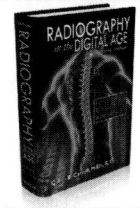

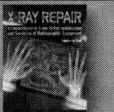

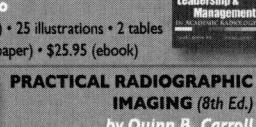

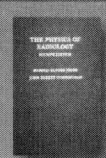